Bioethics

A Culture War

Edited by
Nicholas C. Lund-Molfese
Michael L. Kelly

UNIVERSITY PRESS OF AMERICA,® INC.
Dallas • Lanham • Boulder • New York • Oxford

Copyright © 2004 by
University Press of America,® Inc.
4501 Forbes Boulevard
Suite 200
Lanham, Maryland 20706
UPA Acquisitions Department (301) 459-3366

PO Box 317
Oxford
OX2 9RU, UK

Library of Congress Control Number: 2004109355
ISBN 0-7618-2918-0 (paperback : alk. ppr.)

Contents

Contents

Editor's Note

As the pace of technological development increases, our society finds itself divided in ways that run far deeper than mere political loyalties. Competing notions of health, family, and human dignity have surfaced as a culture war, driving biomedical science into an uncertain future. Modern culture is in great need of people who are willing to bring rigorous ethical thinking to the practice of medicine and health science. The need becomes all the more pressing when the terms of discussion are most often not set by practitioners, but by journalists and interest groups, people more committed to sound-bite discussion than to ethics.

In February 2003, the Integritas Institute of the Archdiocese of Chicago sponsored its second annual conference entitled *Human Dignity and Contemporary Health Science*. The conference once again brought together a distinguished, multi-disciplinary group of scholars to consider recent cultural trends in bioethics, most of them from a Catholic perspective, all of them from a perspective that places the highest value on protecting the dignity of every human life. The essays in this book, with one exception, are the contributions of the conference's participants.

The three sections in this book explore the modern culture war from different perspectives. The first section describes modern cultural notions of health and human suffering. It examines the meaning of suffering in the contemporary world and relates this discussion to the ethical issues surrounding abortion, euthanasia, and the competing conceptions of health. The second section discusses the philosophical origins of the culture war, looking into the problematic bases of various forms of moral relativism and their inadequacy in guiding moral action. The third section contextualizes this abstract discussion in the current political and legal debate about biotechnology, marriage, and the family.

In compiling these essays, it is our intention to present rigorous ethical positions on various pressing issues in the biomedical sciences. We hope to advance a set of moral principles and guidelines that provide an intellectually-sound basis for discussion and debate in the modern culture war. We would like to thank Francis Cardinal George, the Catholic Medical Association, and Fr. Patrick Marshall for their generosity and support.

Introduction

Francis Cardinal George, O.M.I.

This book is an invitation to dialogue. Its contributors seek to add to the great conversation between science and religion and between moral theology and bioethics. The dialogue is rooted in philosophical differences that are quite apart from the facts of a technological science and modern medicine. Two very different understandings of the human person lie at the center of the modern bioethics debate. Much of the importance of this book is to bring into the public domain a view of the human person that is often opposed, ignored, or unacknowledged in our modern culture.

There seem to be two ways of understanding the human person today. On the one hand, some argue that an individual is established by choices rooted in will and, therefore, that moral autonomy is the governing rubric for ethical discussions about biomedical advances. On the other hand, some—and I count myself among them—contend that the human person is first established in a network of relations given by nature and by God; relations that are uncovered in the moral activity each of us undertakes as we grow older; relations that are grown into through a lifetime of freeing oneself from selfishness in order to become ever more generous and self giving, even to the point of self sacrifice.

The relationship between the dignity of human persons (no matter how that dignity is established) and advances in biomedical science turn to a great extent on a point that is often poorly understood: the relationship between freedom and truth. Understood properly, freedom is founded upon truth; it is not a raw, self-defining autonomy. Truth neither restricts personal freedom nor threatens our cherished liberty. In fact, truth promotes freedom and prevents its obstruction. Without knowing the truth about ourselves, we are neither free to make choices nor to understand the purpose of individual freedom, which is the reason that wisdom for the Greeks began with "knowing yourself." In other words, it is not sufficient to know the truth about things as if truth were just regulatory; one must recognize that truth is perfective of the human person. A person who knows the truth is a better person than one who does not. Without this sense of truth as perfective of the human person, one cannot understand the connection between freedom and truth. Objective truth encompasses more than mere physical things; it is also self reflective, involving the truth seeker.

The question of who we are, the question of self-knowledge, is not just an empirical one: how did we come to exist? Nor is it simply a historical question: where do we come from? Nor is it a technical question: what are we able to do? Science and technology offer many answers, fine answers, to these questions, and we must attend to them. But it goes beyond mere theory; it goes beyond ethics as well. The question, "what ought I to do?" does not in itself answer the question, "who am I?"

This is a philosophical and anthropological question that began with the kind of wonder that motivated human beings to reflect upon the world and themselves in philosophical and religious thought. By its very nature, this question has value. It is perfective of the person who is so moved to make the inquiry and who responds to the invitation, given by reality, to fuller self-disclosure and self-discovery.

The individual understanding of the self shapes, in turn, personal integrity. The truth of my statements is measured by my disclosure of the real situation in which I live. However, if I choose to lie or to ignore reality, that too shapes the situation and my self-understanding. This is especially true about painful truths that I may attempt to avoid, for example, when an unwelcome diagnosis forces me to acknowledge the inevitability of my own death. In this instance, I am impelled by truth, and yet I am not forced in the way natural phenomenon are forced, in the way a lighted match forces the ignition of gasoline. Rather, I am free before these kinds of self-revelations to either accept or reject reality and my own moral responsibility, and it takes a certain courage to admit the truth and accept responsibility for my actions. That is the work of freedom. If I have the courage to face such painful situations, I feel a certain satisfaction or liberation, even a certain fullness, perfection, or completion in the midst of that pain. The truth is not simply normative or regulative, it is perfective of my very being as a human person. The truth "sets us free", as Jesus said, a point that can never be overemphasized.

In this sense, human life is not ultimately subject to any physical law. There is freedom to choose right and wrong, a conscious decision to either accept or reject a moral order. There is a whole dimension of embodiment that clearly goes beyond the physical, and it is this dimension that modern medical science tends to ignore.

Our spiritual being seems so familiar that it is easily overlooked. It depends neither upon faith nor esoteric argument. In reading this introduction, most of you are exerting energy as I do in writing it. And, no matter how interesting this subject may be, eventually you will grow tired and your physical energy will be depleted. But, in fact, something additional is going on in this kind of dialogue, and it is remarkable enough that even in great universities this basic truth is left unattended. In conversation, something happens that is more than a loss of mere physical energy. The exchange of ideas is not at all a physical transaction in which energy passes from writer to reader. It is not the same kind of transaction as when you push away a heavy weight, pull a car out of the mud, or spend your morning shoveling the snow. In those instances, you lose energy as you transfer physical power from yourself to the object of your attention. In contrast, the exchange of ideas involves no loss of the idea itself; we engage in communication without loss.

The medieval schoolmen drew attention to this feature of knowing, calling it an immanent operation, an indwelling activity, one that remains in the knower even though there is an exchange. The wonder, however, is that, while it remains in the knower, it is also passed on to another and becomes present to the reader or listener, to the degree of the writer or speaker's clarity and reader or listener's attentiveness. This is the law of the spiritual activity of knowing and communicating, which is immediately available to our experience if we attend to it.

But, there is still more to be gleaned from this ordinary activity of coming to know who we are so that we may live freely as we are created. The philosopher Hegel noted that consciousness has the ability of going out to the other, of identifying with another and returning to oneself all the while retaining one's own identity, all of this without loss. In going out to the object in the act of identifying it and understanding it however superficially, impartially, or inadequately, the mind does not intrude upon the other, it remains what it is. Knowing as distinct from mere thinking occurs only when we are present to the thing as it really is. And here we can only wonder all the more, for we see that we have a relationship, for example, to a classroom and to the objects in it, which is different from the physical relationship by which the chair adjusts itself to our weight or we bump into tables or fall on the floor.

We intuitively think about our knowledge of the room as putting images or ideas in our heads. It is true that we do retain residual ideas, images, and memory once we have left the classroom. But, in actually knowing something, we do not put ideas in our heads as though we are placing pictures in a miniature gallery. Rather, our actual knowing of the classroom puts us into the space in a non-physical way. I, for the sake of argument, am at the same time physically both in a classroom and in my body. In my awareness of my presence in a room, I have now entered into a different form of presence in and to the room. And this should give us pause in answering who we are, because we cannot be free without understanding our environment and the nature of its relationship to us. In so far as we know the objects in this room in some fashion, we do not really put them into our heads. On the contrary, we are cast out into the room in a new, distinct, and wondrous way. In so far as we know the objects, we do not bump into them in our heads, just as we do not upset tables in thinking about them, but we are still truly present to them.

The wonder of knowing and the way in which the operation of knowing discloses something about ourselves allows one to come to a self-knowledge in coming to know anything scientifically; and that knowing is a perfection of my being, which enables me to be free and not simply another object in the classroom like a chalkboard or an eraser. Our knowing is therefore not governed by the justly famous three laws of physics. Knowing is immanent in the person, it is not invasive in the thing known, and it comes about by our submitting ourselves in mind to the way that things really are. The value of truth governs our knowing. Even painful truth brings enrichment, and therefore it is better to know the truth than not to know it; it is more perfective of the human being. Only in knowing thyself, even when it is painful, can I be said to be free. Truth is not only normative, it is perfective.

In the very center of the human person, the spiritual source that is governed and perfected by truth, we come upon the secret of human freedom and the bond between freedom and truth. It is no wonder, then, that truth has the power to attract and convict us. Truth opens us up to ourselves, to others, and to the world. Truth is the power that draws us out of the deadening passivity of a purely physical existence; an existence that would otherwise lack the medium of a genuinely personal spiritual life, the life of freedom.

I make this point because it is so often lost not only in scientific discussion, in the strict sense, but even in discussions such as this. If we are to come to a dialogue, we have to clarify the basis of who is dialoguing so that we can know the truth; and the truth will set us free.

A last word about our social situation today: it is a troubling paradox that both freedom and human dignity, which underwrites freedom, should be threatened in a functioning democratic society. In fact, to quote Leon Kass, "human dignity is at risk from an alliance between democracy and ethical relativism, which removes any stable moral reference point from political and social life . . . And which challenges our self understanding as creatures of dignity rendering us incapable of recognizing dangers to our humanity."[1]

These are dangers that arise from a purely reductive science that puts enormous power into our hands. It leaves us without a common meaning and purpose, and ultimately fails to represent the organic human body as an animated, purposive, and striving being. I thank the Integritas Institute for this opportunity to know ourselves and the world more thoroughly in order to improve our understanding of human freedom.

NOTE

1. Kass, Leon, *Life, Liberty, and the Defense of Dignity: The Challenge for Bioethics.* (San Francisco, Encounter Books, 2002), p. 20.

I

A MODERN CULTURE WAR: HEALTH AND HUMAN SUFFERING

1

What is the Culture War About?[1]

Nicholas C. Lund-Molfese

I. INTRODUCTION

The ubiquitous phrase, "Americans are deeply divided" appears to be an obligatory prefix to much of the media's reporting on the most controversial issues in contemporary bioethics.[2] That reputable opinion polls of Americans demonstrate a division of opinion on the "life issues" of abortion, embryo experimentation, cloning and euthanasia—and that these opinions are deeply held—is beyond doubt.

More important than acknowledging the existence of a division of popular opinion is the undertaking of ascertaining its meaning. It is to this task which this paper endeavors to attend. I do not take up this assignment with any pretensions to neutrality, but with a specific purpose in mind: advancing the gospel of life through the tools of the social sciences in the context of our current cultural situation.

That a false answer to the question, "What is the culture war really about?" cannot serve my purpose is self evident, but it is no less the case that some valid answers are of greater practical importance than others. The question itself has no shortage of competing answers and on any list of leading candidates would be: the nature of the family,[3] the judicial usurpation of politics,[4] and the sexual revolution.[5] Undoubtedly, our cultural divisions are "about" a mixture of issues and each way of answering the question, each description of the common root underlying our disagreements over these issues, privileges some aspect over others. Out of the many proposed answers, I have selected two (based on their helpfulness and importance for the fulfillment of my purpose) for discussion in the next section of this paper.

3

II. WHAT IS THE CULTURE WAR REALLY ABOUT?

The Culture War is a Spiritual Battle Between the Devil and Humanity

In, *How to Win the Culture War: A Christian Battle Plan for a Society in Crisis*, Professor Peter Kreeft of Boston College's philosophy department, looks at our situation from the theological perspective of an evangelical-Catholic.[6] He characterizes what is at stake as a war in which "[o]ur enemies are demons, Fallen Angels, Evil spirits" and also our own sinfulness.[7] The solution is for more of us to become saints.[8] The "culture war" reflected in the sociologists' polls is really an epiphenomenon of the spiritual warfare that is particularly intense in our time. Kreeft believes that the private revelation of Pope Leo XIII provides "the most reasonable hypothesis".[9] In Leo's vision, he sees Satan choose the twentieth century as the century, in all of human history, that he will most afflict the human race. It was in response to this vision that Leo composed the well-known "Prayer to Saint Michael."[10]

Kreeft does not leave his readers at the level of ultimate cause, but rather, goes on to trace the multitude of proximate causes of American culture's corruption which flow from this demonic affliction: disbelief in the existence of Satan; ecclesial decadence; the division of Christianity; the perceived opposition between virtues (e.g. love vs. truth); relativism; and the sexual revolution with its resultant weakening of the family.[11] Regarding this last point, Kreeft remarks, "we cannot win the culture war unless we win the sex war, because sex is the effective religion of our culture, and religion is the strongest force in the world, the strongest motivation there is."[12]

What then is Kreeft's answer to the question, "What is the culture war really about?" At its foundation, it is the result of the actions and afflictions of the devil upon the twentieth century. Licentiousness is the preferred tool of the evil one in corrupting society and building the culture of death. The cause of the culture's corruption is placed, to a substantial degree, outside of itself. While the healing of the culture will have legal and sociological components, it is primarily a matter of spiritual warfare. In the context of contemporary American culture, many will see talk of "spiritual warfare" as indistinguishable from an invitation to "religious warfare," but nothing could be farther from Kreeft's intent. He makes clear that the enemy is not other persons who disagree with him—they are the culture war's victims—it is Evil itself that is the enemy.

For an orthodox Christian believer, Kreeft's analysis is surely instructive and edifying. The weapons of the spirit, the spiritual means of prayer and fasting, are the most powerful means available to us. Saints are, even by secular standards, among the most influential persons in the history of western civilization. Kreeft reminds us of what is of ultimate importance and also of who is the true enemy of humanity. This is a helpful accomplishment. Most importantly, the implication of his thesis is that, however persuasive, arguments or political-legal maneuvers alone will not be sufficient to win the culture war. As I will propose in the third section of this paper, for many people, faith will be required before morally upright decisions in the context of abortion and euthanasia appear as realistic options for choice.

The Culture War is a Confusion Over Sacredness

Another scholar, from a very different perspective, who believes that religious/spiritual notions are at the heart of our cultural disagreements, is New York University law professor Ronald Dworkin. His 1993 book, *Life's Dominion: An Argument about Abortion, Euthanasia, and Individual Freedom*,[13] was received rapturously by the American cultural elites—at least if the front and back cover blurbs on his book are to be believed. For example, *The New York Times Book Review* called it a "wonderfully rich and evocative [book] . . . brimming with insights" and a "masterpiece" which was "a feast for the mind and a balm for the soul." *The Boston Globe*'s reviewer offers that, "I wish there were a way to make sure that this book found its way into the hands and minds of those people of good faith who stand on opposite sides of the abortion issue."

The fact that Dworkin's book found a ready audience among some partisans of the culture wars was appropriate. It was his intention that by offering a different explanation of our culture's debate over the life issues "it would allow Americans to "find a collective solution to the political controversy that all sides could accept with dignity."[14] The "dignified" solution proposed by Dworkin, however, is indistinguishable from those proposed by Planned Parenthood or End-of-Life Choices (formerly, The Hemlock Society), or, for that matter, the editorial pages of the *New York Times* and *Boston Globe*.

Dworkin spends most of the book offering a defense of the constitutional validity of the Supreme Court's majority opinions creating (*Roe v. Wade*)[15] and upholding (*Planned Parenthood v. Casey*)[16] a constitutional right to abortion. A good chunk of the remainder is an exercise in sociology focused on the intriguing discrepancies in public opinion on abortion and the right to life. For example, polls indicate that most people think that abortion ends a human life; however, polls also show that a large majority favors abortion being legal in "hard cases" such as instances of rape and incest.[17]

Dworkin reconciles the data by positing that pro-lifers are confused regarding their own beliefs. They cannot really believe their own stated position: that the unborn are full human persons in the same sense as, for example, any twelve year old. If pro-lifers truly believed their own arguments, they could not support abortion in the hard cases.[18] According to Dworkin, the best way to make sense of the data is to view the pro-life position as the avowal of the proposition that human life is sacred. This principle is universally affirmed, including by those in favor of legal abortion.[19] For example, according to this line of argument, persons who are pro-choice are defending the sacredness of life when they support the right of a woman, pregnant with an unwanted child, to have an abortion. In this context, the termination of her pregnancy is a defense of the sacredness of her own life. The "great abortion debate," thus, is a spiritual debate over the meaning and priority of different ways of weighing the sacred.[20]

Dworkin's explanation for the source of the culture war—the entire pro-life movement is an intellectual confusion—is more a statement of prejudice than a plausible argument. To claim that prominent pro-life intellectuals, of which there are too many to cite, are either liars or confused requires an extraordinary level of contempt for one's interlocutors. There are those who are motivated by reason, and thus agree with him, and then there are "the motives that drive many enemies of freedom of choice [which] are too deep—too unexamined, unreasoned, and visceral—to respond to argument at all."[21] Bigotry aside, Dworkin does raise an important fact to prominence in the course of his book: the apparent logical incongruity displayed in public opinion on abortion is of more than passing significance. I will propose an alternative analysis of the importance of this discrepancy in this paper's next section.

III. THE PROXIMATE CAUSE OF OUR CULTURAL WAR IS A FALSE UNDERSTANDING OF SUFFERING.

"For suffering, Rodion Romanovitch, is a great thing."
—Fyodor Dostoevsky[22]

When the meaning of human suffering is misunderstood, the result is not merely unfortunate, it is disastrous. A false understanding of suffering generates a false compassion, a tenderness that kills. As Walker Percy has one of his characters in *The Thanatos Syndrome* teach us:

> Tenderness is the first disguise of the murderer . . . Never in the history of the world have there been so many civilized tenderhearted souls as have lived in this century. . . . More people have been killed in this century by tender hearted souls than by cruel barbarians in all other centuries put together. . . . Do you know where tenderness always leads. . . . To the gas chambers.[23]

The thesis of this paper is that a false cultural understanding of suffering is at the root of popular support for abortion, euthanasia, embryo experimentation and cloning. Each of these elements of the culture of death is an emotionally attractive option for choice, in certain circumstances, based on the hope of alleviating or preventing suffering. As the issues involved in each of these four cases are similar and as we have more data regarding abortion and euthanasia, I will focus my attention on these two and assert that a similar analysis could validly be done regarding the remaining issues. By the end of this paper I hope to have demonstrated that, as long as suffering is perceived as the greatest evil, we can expect legal scholars and the general public to continue to justify the killing of the unborn and the elderly under the guise of compassion and tenderheartedness.

Abortion as a Solution to Suffering

Annually, approximately 1.3 million women have an abortion in the United States.[24] Over 25% of all pregnant women chose to have an abortion rather than continue their pregnancy to term.[25] When asked why, 20% of women who have an abortion cite inadequate finances, 32% cite not being mature enough to raise a child and 24% stated that they did not desire another child or that the birth of another child at this time would be too disruptive in their life. The remainder mentioned a diversity of reasons (fetal defect, 3%, women's health 3%, rape or incest 1% and other 4%).[26]

While abortion (and euthanasia) is categorized as "a problem," when examined from the perspective of the social sciences, it can also be viewed as "a solution" from the perspective of individuals who chose them. Abortion is not chosen for itself. No one (unless engaged in a pathological form of self-abuse) sets out to get pregnant in order that they may have an abortion. A woman who is pregnant and does not desire the birth of an additional child for one of the above reasons has a limited number of choices open to her. Faced with the fact of not being mature enough to be a parent or lacking the financial resources to take care of a child—let alone the emotions involved in being pregnant by rape—a woman can anticipate the suffering that will result from choosing to carry the child to term.[27]

If a woman chooses, from the options available to her, based on which choice will bring about the least future anticipated suffering, she will not (in a limited sense) unreasonably see abortion as an attractive option for choice in many situations. The variations in public support for the legal availability of abortion, which I will examine in detail shortly, exactly track the perceived "suffering calculus." Support is greatest in cases such as rape and incest where Americans believe that carrying the child to term will result in the greatest burden, the greatest suffering, on the women involved. Situations and stories, like the one that follows, which implicitly argue for abortion as a solution to avoid great suffering, are an essential reason for what support exists among the American people for maintaining the legality of abortion.

The Power of a Story and of the Hard Cases

In 1992, the story of Sherri Finkbine[28] and the events of her life were awarded the highest recognition our celebrity-obsessed society grants—a full length HBO special starring Sissy Spacek and a cast of notables. The film, "A Private Matter," makes no pretense at neutrality but is "shamelessly pro-choice" according to one of its producers.[29] It chronicles Finkbine's ulti-mately successful efforts in 1962 to abort her fifth child after she found out that the thalidomide in the painkillers she took was known to cause birth de-fects. Panicked at the thought of having to take care of a "horribly" deformed child, she went to her family doctor who, along with her husband, agreed that a "therapeutic" abortion was advisable and arrangements were made at a nearby hospital. Then, for reasons that remain unclear, but perhaps in an effort to further the pro-choice cause, she decided to tell her story to a re-porter for a local newspaper.

The hospital, in response to the growing publicity, reversed itself and refused to provide the abortion because doing so might subject it to crim-inal liability. At this point, Finkbine's situation became a national sensa-tion and received repeated coverage in many of the nation's major news-papers. Ultimately, she went to Sweden where she was finally successful in securing the abortion she so desired. During the ensuing public debate she garnered considerable popular sympathy and was depicted by the media as the perfect wife and mother. As the host of a local television sta-tion's *Romper Room* show and the devoted mother of four children, she cut a sympathetic image in the popular imagination. She later explained that she did not want a disabled child who might not have either arms or legs and who might "sit in the park and have people give him peanuts and things. Had it not been for the abortion, I would have [had to] take care of the four children I had, and the head and torso [referring to her aborted child]."[30]

How important are "hard case" stories like Finkbine's to public support for abortion? Clearly these are the cases that the pro-choice movement prefers to focus on. When Sarah Weddington, lead plaintiff's attorney in *Roe v. Wade*, met Finkbine years after her abortion she said: "It's a privilege to meet you. If it hadn't been for you, my job ten years later would have been much more difficult."[31] This was no mere flattery by Weddington. In *Closed Cham-bers*, Edward Lazarus, former Supreme Court clerk to Justice Harry Black-mun, the author of the majority opinion in *Roe v. Wade*, says of Finkbine's saga:

> This highly publicized ordeal, of a suburban housewife and mother terrified of giving birth to a terribly malformed child, placed the idea of therapeutic abor-tion in a sympathetic and easily imaginable context and brought home to many Americans the need for abortion law reform.[32]

In addition, Planned Parenthood Federation of America, Inc. lists the thalido-mide-caused birth defects and Finkbine's well-publicized quest for an abortion on their website timeline "Family Planning in America."[33]

The importance and power of so-called hard cases in shaping public opinion in support of legalized abortion should not be underestimated. Clearly those favoring a legal "right to choose" abortion never fail to keep in the foremost of public thought relatively rare, exceptional situations such as rape, incest, fetal deformity and threat to the life of the mother—situations which collectively motivate no more than seven percent of all abortions performed annually.[34] The reasoning behind this emphasis is flawless. These are the cases in which, poll after poll demonstrates, the pro-choice forces win over the majority of Americans.

Pro-lifers cannot just ignore these relatively rare hard cases, because their impact is much greater than their numbers. These cases are disproportionately effective in undermining the development of a pro-life majority in America. This is because opposing abortion in the hard cases means accepting extreme suffering, suffering for which the public sees abortion as the only solution.

This is a good point to return to the insight of Ronald Dworkin, already discussed, regarding the importance of the apparent logical discrepancies in polling data regarding abortion. The data is not without ambiguity and some scholars dispute both Dworkin's interpretation and the importance he gives these statistics.[35] While I reject his interpretation, I concur in his judgment that there is something deserving of our attention here.

Dworkin focuses on four different polls: one conducted by the Gallup polling organization in 1991 and commissioned by Americans United for Life, a 1990 Wirthlin poll funded by the United States Conference of Catholic Bishops, a 1992 *Time*/CNN poll and a 1992 NBC News/*Wall Street Journal* poll.[36] A little later in his text he brings in a fifth, a 1980 *New York Times*/CBS News poll.[37] Among the statistics he cites are: Abortion is just as bad as killing a person who has already been born, it is murder (36.8%); Abortion is not murder, but it does involve the taking of human life (28.3%); All human life, including that of the unborn, should be protected (60%); A woman should be able to get an abortion . . . no matter what the reason (49%); The life of the unborn should be protected (60%); Abortion should be illegal in all circumstances (7%); Abortion should be legal only when necessary to save the mother's life (14%).[38]

Collectively, Dworkin finds these results "baffling" but never-the-less is able to reconcile the data by concluding that persons who condemn abortion do so in a "detached" manner. By detached, he means that, however strongly some people may believe that abortion is murder, they also "really" believe (if they really understood what they believe) that the decision to have an abortion must be left to the individual woman.[39] However,

Dworkin's conclusion regarding the beliefs of ordinary people seems even more baffling than the putative problem he is attempting to solve. How many ordinary people believe that rape, racism or infanticide is wrong in a "detached" way? Real people are detached about what condiments they put on their burger, not matters of life and death. Categorizing our beliefs on abortion as "religious" and raising abortion to the level of a sacrament doesn't detach people of good will from love of neighbor. It is that love which forbids detachment, which is to say indifference, in the face of injustice to one's brothers and sisters.

The alternative I offer is that the data Dworkin cites can be taken to demonstrate that people's opinions on abortion are more sophisticated, and more deeply thought-through, than the blunt instruments used in these polls can measure. More helpful than asking people about abortion in general is to ask very specific questions about abortion in certain categories of cases. This gives greater insight into what is really at issue in the responses received. For that, we need to turn to a different set of polling data.

The National Right to Life Committee maintains a detailed account of polling data on its web site. Most helpful, for my purposes, are the detailed questions asked in a November 1994 Wirthlin poll. According to Wirthlin, only nine percent of Americans favor prohibiting abortion in all circumstances, the same percentage that favors not prohibiting any abortions for any reason. Another eleven percent would permit abortion only when the mother's life was at risk. In contrast, the vast majority, **seventy-four percent**, believed, at a minimum, that abortion should be legal, for at least the first three months, in cases of rape or incest or to save the mother's life.[40] The pro-life position loses badly in the court of public opinion when these exceptional cases are made central to the abortion debate and thus they have an importance far exceeding their relative frequency. This is the real importance of the inconsistencies considered by Dworkin. Why do we feel it is ok to kill the unborn in cases of rape? Is it because in those cases we have less solidarity with the "product of the rape?"

Suffering Misunderstood: Killing as a Solution to Suffering

The formulation of an effective response to this state of affairs must begin with an examination of the root causes of public support for legalized abortion in exceptional circumstances. What causes Americans, who are opposed to most abortions—presumably because they believe that abortion is the taking of a human life—to think that abortion should be legally permitted when the child is conceived as a result of rape or incest? What caused the huge outpouring of sympathy for Sherri Finkbine's decision to kill her disabled unborn child, a child who was merely *at risk* of being born without any arms or legs?

A related phenomenon can be seen in the *de facto*, if not yet *de jure*, near legalization of infanticide, at least when committed by the victim's mother. For some reason perpetrators of this form of "domestic violence" receive lighter sentences for first degree murder than most drunk drivers. For example, the widely reported story of a Canadian woman who shot a pellet from an air gun into the brain of her unborn child provoked little public outcry—even when the Canadian courts ruled that she could not be convicted of any crime. Miraculously, the child was born alive a few days later and appeared to be in good heath after doctors operated on him and removed the projectile.[41]

Amanda Beckett, 18, got a mere one-and-a-half years in prison for killing her son and placing him in the trash.[42] Melissa Drexler was sentenced to 15 years in prison for drowning her baby boy in the toilet bowl at her senior prom, but is likely to be out of prison in as little as three years with time off for good behavior.[43] In the case of the infamous New Jersey couple who rented a hotel room in Delaware, beat their newborn son to death, stuffed him in a garbage bag and tossed him into the trash—mom got a mere two-and-one-half years while dad was sentenced to two years in jail.[44] Finally, there is the story of Marie Noe of Philadelphia who pled guilty to killing eight of her children with her own hands and placing the blame on Sudden Infant Death Syndrome. What punishment did the court deem fitting for this mass murder? She received a sentence of probation and five years of home confinement. She will never see the inside of a prison.[45]

To use a political slogan from a bygone national election, *where is the outrage?* If we do not exactly approve of the conduct of these women, at least we "understand" the difficulty of the situation they faced—and I do not intend to make light of the serious suffering and misfortune of these parent-murderers. To have a baby as an unmarried teenager with, as in some of these cases, little family or community support, takes great courage.[46] In the same way, most parents can sympathize with the sufferings and difficulties facing Sherri Finkbine. Any parent of a child with a serious disability can tell you of the sufferings they have had to face and the difficulties placed on the entire family.[47] It takes little imagination to gain an understanding, however limited, of the suffering involved in carrying to term a child conceived by rape or continuing with a pregnancy that resulted from being forced into sex by a family member.[48] Our culture understands the sufferings these persons experience, all the while completely misunderstanding the nature of suffering.

Likewise, the woman who seeks an abortion due to some serious difficulty caused by her pregnancy, or the mother and/or father who kill their child soon after birth, are often acting in a situation of great suffering or great expected future suffering. There are abortions of nothing more than convenience, but in the "hard cases" of rape or incest, it is mere callousness to deny the human reality that the pregnant woman is experiencing. Often in these cases **abortion or infanticide is chosen as a solution to suffering** by the distraught parent. They are acting out of a cultural misunderstanding of the nature and meaning of suffering.

According to our culture, suffering is first of all meaningless and second of all perceived as the greatest evil. It is meaningless in that, in a world without God, human suffering is not ultimately explicable. Life is reduced to a balancing act of pain and pleasure in which suffering is to be avoided at any cost and by any method, be it abortion, euthanasia, or infanticide. There has even developed substantial popular approval for abortion, and to a lesser extent infanticide, as morally praiseworthy choices where such killing is perceived as necessary to end present, or to prevent future, suffering. Thus, killing a disabled child before birth becomes a "compassionate" choice or "the best choice in a difficult situation." Before killing his wife, two children, and ultimately himself, Mark Barton of Atlanta left a note for police explaining his actions: "I killed the children to exchange for them five minutes of pain for a lifetime of pain. I forced myself to do it to keep them from suffering so much later."[49]

Euthanasia as a Solution to Suffering

"In the absence of this faith now, we govern by tenderness. It is a tenderness which, long since cut off from the person of Christ, is wrapped in theory. When tenderness is detached from the source of tenderness, its logical outcome is terror. It ends in forced labor camps and in the fumes of the gas chamber."[50]

Flannery O'Connor, from "Mystery and Manners"

Since the 1997 legalization of physician assisted suicide in Oregon, the number of assisted suicides has totaled 129 "patient" deaths, with 38 of that number taking place in 2002.[51] Within the legal and political debate that surrounded the enactment of the law we can see quite clearly the attitude that suffering is meaningless and to be avoided at all costs, even at the price of intentionally killing oneself or another person. From this perspective, as we shall see, suffering gives one both a moral and a legal right to death.

On October 27, 1997, physician-assisted suicide became a legal, medical solution to the problem of suffering for the residents of Oregon. This was the conclusion of a long legal and political battle that began with the introduction of Measure 16, "The Oregon Death with Dignity Act." The Act was a citizens' initiative passed by the voters of Oregon by a margin of 51% to 49% in November of 1994, but its legal effect was delayed by court-imposed injunctions for almost three years. In November of 1997 the state legislature gave the voters of Oregon an opportunity to change their mind. Oregon House Bill 2954 placed Measure 51 on the general election ballot. The measure, which was defeated by a margin of 60% to 40%, would have repealed Measure 16.[52]

Oregon law requires that the state's Department of Human Services collect and disseminate information on the implementation of the Death with Dignity act. The department's 2002 annual report informs us of how long the "patients" took to die (three took six hours and one took fourteen) and what reasons they gave for choosing to end their life: "losing autonomy," 84%; a "decreasing ability to participate in activities that made life enjoyable," 84%; "losing control of bodily functions," 47%; "burden on family," 37%; "inadequate pain control," 26%; "financial implications," 3% (totals do not add up to 100% because patients can identify more than one reason).[53] These reasons are fears about future anticipated suffering. In choosing suicide, 38 persons chose death over enduring suffering. Morally, there is an inexact parallel of these 38 separate personal decisions to the collective decision of 60% of Oregon voters to keep suicide as an available option for choice as a solution to their own (or others) anticipated future suffering.

Not only is physician assisted suicide legal in Oregon, the state also pays for the "service" to be performed for the poor. Since 1998 the state has covered physician assisted suicide in its Medicaid program.[54] Oregon not only offers financially assisted suicide to the poor, but it also rations health care to Medicaid beneficiaries using a utilitarian prioritization formula. A "Health Services Commission" examines all illnesses and the treatments available and prioritizes them based on their cost effectiveness. The most recent version of the "Prioritized List of Health Services," released October 1, 2003, contains 730 items; however, there was only enough funding granted by the legislature to cover the 549 most cost-effective treatments.[55] Persons without health insurance who lack the financial means to pay for the 181 uncovered procedures out of their own pocket must simply go without medical care.

Apparently assisted suicide is very cost effective as it sits at No. 265 on the list, euphemistically listed as "Comfort Care." That is higher than "Treatable Cancer of the Colon" (No. 273) and way above "Endometriosis" (No. 496) and "Cancer of the Liver, Treatable" (No. 501) but not too far ahead of "Induced Abortion" (No. 300). What treatments did not get covered? "Cystic Acne" (No. 554) just missed and "Acute Anal Fissures" at No. 625 didn't even come close. As one might expect, persons who have unfunded diseases are, as *Slate* magazine puts it:

> irate that a lifesaving operation in the territory around No. 570 can depend on the annual appropriating whims of the legislature, while a free barbiturate consolation prize is safely ensconced at No. [265]. Defenders of the commission counter that it would be unconscionable to deny the poor a right as fundamental as death.[56]

What caused Oregon voters to choose assisted suicide, twice, as a solution to the problem of suffering? The Catholic Church and other churches in Oregon did their best to present an alternative vision of the meaning of suffering, but it is fair to say that their vision was twice rejected by the voters of Oregon. Opponents of the measure repeatedly pointed to the religious motivation of many of those opposed to physician-assisted suicide. In addition, the author of the original Measure 16, Barbara Coombs Lee, made references to "the dictates of the pope" in her speeches, and several different television advertisements targeted the Catholic Church by name.[57]

After two lively debates on the issue, it is difficult to argue the voters were misinformed or that they did not know what they were voting for. The obvious answer is that the majority of the voters chose for death and against Christianity's understanding of suffering. Such a choice is more than another milestone in the culture war. The language of the social sciences, of polls and politics, is simply inadequate. It is in this context that Peter Kreeft's description of our situation, examined at the start of this paper, as a battle between humanity and the Evil One, shines as the only adequate characterization. The situation in Oregon was not imposed on the people by a few unelected judges as in the case of abortion, but freely chosen by the electorate. As such, it represents a unique instance of the advance of the culture of death where an entire political society, one of the fifty states, has embraced death. In this situation, believing Christians cannot help but see in this cultural conflict a more-than-human source of evil at work which will require a more than human effort to combat it successfully.

IV. THE MEANING OF SUFFERING

Cultural attitudes towards suffering determine, perhaps more than any other single factor, a given society's support for what John Paul II calls "the culture of death." I have argued that a desire to avoid suffering is among the chief forces leading people to choose abortion and euthanasia. On this point, the noted Catholic moral theologian, Germain Grisez, offers the following insight:

> The extent of the abuses of biomedical technologies suggests that the wrongful options are very appealing. Why is that? Human beings exist in a fallen condition. . . . In this fallen situation, choosing uprightly often seems impractical. Lacking hope for any happiness beyond death, people go after what they imagine might make them happy during this life.[58]

As long as many of our fellow citizens "lack hope for any happiness beyond death" can we really expect to make progress in the cultural acceptance of the value of life? Can a merely human philosophy or reasoned arguments reverse our current situation? I concur with the implicitly negative answer to this question given by Peter Kreeft. Only if the Christian mystery of suffering is accepted will abortion and euthanasia be clearly seen for what they are, false choices for death and against life. Sin, not suffering, is the greatest evil, but that truth is simply incommunicable to the majority of people in our culture who do not understand the true nature of suffering. Conveying the truth of suffering is one of the essential tasks for evangelization in our time. However, it is no surprise that, where there is a crucial need, we find Pope John Paul II stepping forward.

It is to John Paul II's 1984 Apostolic Letter, *Salvifici Doloris*[59] (On the Christian Meaning of Human Suffering), called by the respected Protestant philosopher Alvin Plantinga, "one of the finest documents (outside the Bible) ever written on this topic," that we must turn for the adequate means of addressing the advancing culture of death.[60] He teaches that suffering is not only "inseparable from man's earthly existence," (§3) it is somehow "essential to the nature of man" and "belongs to man's transcendence." (§2) As man's earthly life is always "on the long path of suffering," and as the Church was "born of the mystery of Redemption in the cross of Christ," suffering is a privileged meeting place between man and the Church so that man-in-his-suffering "becomes the way for the Church." (§3)

This teaching stands in sharp contrast to our culture's perception that suffering is evil in itself and to be avoided by any means, even the killing of the innocent. Rather, the Pope teaches that while suffering entered the world due to human sin, it has a new meaning in light of the redemptive work of Christ. Suffering "is present in the world in order to release love" and "in order to transform the whole of human civilization into a 'civilization of love.'" (§30) Every person is called to participate in that suffering through which our redemption was accomplished and through which all suffering was redeemed. "In bringing about the Redemption through suffering, Christ has also raised human suffering to the level of the Redemption. Thus each man in his suffering can also become a sharer in the redemptive suffering of Christ." (§19) Christ, who took on all human suffering, participates in every individual's suffering and that suffering is "capable of being infused with the same power of God manifested in Christ's Cross." (§23)

One could not imagine a greater contrast between our cultures' understanding of suffering and the teaching of the Magisterium. Once more, John Paul II holds forth with confidence in the beauty of the Bride of Christ, even on what one otherwise might think was the field of battle most disadvantageous to her: suffering and the problem of evil. Judging by appearances, suffering is one of the chief causes of atheism and of dissent against the teachings of the Church. In *The Problem of Pain*[61], C. S. Lewis, recalling his attitude before his conversion to Christianity, lists the various aspects of human suffering, including war, disease, terror, and the emptiness of the universe. He then concludes:

> If you asked me to believe that this was the work of a benevolent and omnipotent spirit, I [would] reply that all the evidence points in the opposite direction. Either there is no spirit behind the universe, or else a spirit indifferent to good and evil, or else an evil spirit.[62]

Lewis, being a serious thinker, was eventually able to see through the problem of evil; however, others have not been as fortunate. The problem of evil has various formulations, but Alice von Hildebrand's phrasing captures the aspect that the Pope is primarily interested in addressing. Hildebrand writes:

> When a person, confronting the intensity of real suffering, raises the question in despair; "How can God who is both infinitely good and infinitely powerful permit such tortures?", we face an insoluble mystery. Faith, however, can shed light upon it. . . . Any ray of light shed on this mystery is bound to be a blessing for suffering humanity. On the other hand, the conviction that suffering is meaningless is bound to throw men into a state of revolt and despair.[63]

Thus, the first principle of a Christian understanding of suffering is **that suffering is meaningful**—meaningful on the most ultimate level—the level of salvation. This perhaps explains John Paul II's confidence. The personal experience of suffering demands an adequate answer and only the Church can provide that answer in its fullness. Therefore, the universal personal experience of suffering provides a unique opportunity for the Church to bring man closer to God. A comparison between the theology of suffering offered by the Church and the solutions to suffering offered by our culture (euthanasia and abortion) illustrates the superiority of the Church's Magisterium as an answer to the universally experienced problem of suffering.

As John Paul II notes in *Salvifici Doloris*, human persons suffer in a variety of ways, including physical suffering and moral suffering. Physical suffering denotes the body as the primary locus of the suffering while moral suffering "is a pain of the soul." There is a psychological dimension to each of these kinds of suffering, but neither one is identical with the psychological aspect of the human person. Moral or spiritual suffering has not been studied to the same degree as physical suffering, which the medical sciences examine, but it is no less diverse or complex. (§5) What modern medicine has done in the way of cataloging and specifying physical illness, the Scriptures, in part, do for spiritual suffering. (§6)

But what is the meaning and nature of suffering? The endurance of suffering is passive; man is the subject acted upon by suffering. A person may respond to suffering with various psychological movements such as sadness, or disappointment; however, suffering remains essentially passive. Within the psychological dimension of each experience of suffering, "there is always an experience of evil, which causes the individual to suffer." Thus the existence or ultimate cause of suffering can only be explained by reference to evil. (§7)

It is important to note that the Pope does not call suffering evil in itself.[64] Suffering is caused by evil in that we undergo suffering when we are aware of evil, but suffering is not itself evil. Later in his Apostolic Letter, the Pope will go on to say: ". . . suffering has special value in the eyes of the Church. It is something good . . ." (§24). Aquinas, in the course of answering the question "Whether Bodily Pain is the Greatest Evil?" states that: "now pain or sorrow for that which is truly evil cannot be the greatest evil, for there is something worse, namely either not to reckon as evil that which is really evil, or not to reject it."[65]

Suffering is knowledge of evil but is not evil in itself. Frequently its existence serves as a helpful spiritual or physical warning that something is amiss. Physical pain is often the first sign of a serious illness; it informs us that something has gone wrong and that we need medical assistance. Likewise, spiritual sufferings, such as "pangs of conscience," frequently prompt reflection and repentance. Of course, sometimes we become aware of evil but are unable to do anything about the situation; one might receive a phone call that one's child has died or that one's spouse is gravely ill. Such information naturally and appropriately causes great suffering. Even here, the evil is not in our knowledge of a certain state of affairs but in the state of affairs themselves. While we experience our knowledge of these evils as suffering, the knowledge itself remains a basic good.

"Salvation means liberation from evil." (§14) Christ liberates man from sin by means of His cross, that is, by the means of suffering. The work of salvation is a labor of suffering. (§16) Every person is called to participate personally in that suffering through which our redemption was accomplished and through which all suffering was redeemed. "In bringing about the Redemption through suffering, Christ has also raised human suffering to the level of the Redemption. Thus each man in his suffering can also become a sharer in the redemptive suffering of Christ." (§19) Christ, who took on all human suffering, participates in every individual's suffering.

Suffering (the Cross) is the one universal door through which all must pass to enter the kingdom of God. (§21) While on the human level suffering is an "emptying," on the divine level it is a glorifying or a "filling up" and an invitation to manifest the "moral greatness of man." The glory of suffering can be seen not only in the martyrs, but also in those who, while not believing in Christ, "suffer and give their lives for the truth." (§22) The Pope explains that:

> The weaknesses of all human sufferings are capable of being infused with the same power of God manifested in Christ's cross. In such a concept, to suffer

means to become particularly susceptible, particularly open to the working of
the salvific powers of God, offered to humanity in Christ. In Him God has confirmed His desire to act especially through suffering. . . . (§23)

From a Christian perspective, suffering is an opportunity for everyone, Christian and non-believer alike, to experience the power of God and share in the
work of redemption. In the midst of each individual's suffering, Christ is
present to share that person's suffering—just as he invites each of us to share
His suffering. This inter-participation of suffering unites our sufferings and
Christ's sufferings, as well as uniting us with Christ personally.

In the final analysis, the Church's Magisterium teaches that suffering is **a
gift** and **an opportunity**. "It is something good, before which the Church
bows down in reverence with all the depth of her faith in the Redemption."
(§24) Suffering has a power which "draws a person interiorly close to Christ.
. . . It is a vocation."[66] (§26) Further, suffering is infinitely meaningful for it is:

> the irreplaceable mediator and author of the good things which are indispensa-
> ble for the world's salvation. It is suffering, **more than anything else**, which
> clears the way for the grace which transforms human souls. Suffering, **more
> than anything else**, makes present in the history of humanity the powers of
> the Redemption. (§27)

IV. CONCLUSION

The "hard cases" of abortion and euthanasia are not "hard" because the ap-
plication of the relevant exceptionless moral norm—one may never intentionally kill an innocent human person—is unclear, but because the applica-
tion requires the acceptance of suffering. Motivated by the desire to avoid
suffering by any means, persons and societies avail themselves of medical
technologies which violate the dignity of the human person or destroy human life. For example, supporting the prohibition of abortion in cases of
rape requires accepting the foreseeable, but unintended, consequence that a
woman who conceives by rape may suffer emotionally. Finding that suffering unacceptable, a large majority of Americans support the legality of abortion in cases of rape. The situation regarding euthanasia is similar.

In this context, John Paul II's effort to remind our post-Christian culture of
the true meaning of suffering is of enormous social consequence. A principled rejection of suffering as a good drives the modern acceptance of abortion and euthanasia. Suffering is no longer atonement or expiation; a chance
for growth and renewal. It is an empty evil without meaning and, as already
noted, meaningless suffering is one of the most intolerable things a person
can experience. Without God, suffering cannot be anything but meaningless.

There can be nothing greater than the balancing of pain and pleasure because there is nothing greater than individual experience; there is no salvation history of suffering to which one's own experience is a part. For the believing Christian, on the other hand, no one suffers alone, but always with Christ.

Only when suffering is understood in the context of Christ will there be sufficient public support to provide legal protection for human life in "hard cases." Only in such a culture will there be sufficient support for persons to choose life, even in the face of great current or future suffering. There is no culture of life apart from the Gospel of life and there is no Gospel of life without Christ.

NOTES

1. This essay draws on research and analysis previously published in a substantially different form. See, "The Gift of Suffering vs. Euthanasia," *Social Justice Review*, (Vol. 90: Num. 11–12, November/December 1999) and "*Salvifici Doloris*: A Challenge to Catholic Social Scientists," *Social Justice Review*, (Vol. 91: Num. 7–8, July/August, 2000). This essay benefited from extensive editing and citation verification by my co-editor, Michael L. Kelly. While I am grateful for his assistance, any errors that remain are solely my own.

2. An electronic search of major media and other information resources available via Internet revealed 163 usages of the phrase "Americans are deeply divided."

3. Paul T. Mero, "Justices Deliver a Loss for the Family," *The Salt Lake Tribune*, June 29, 2003. Gary Bauer, "Commentary: Losing the Culture War," *Crosswalk.com*, www.crosswalk.com/news/1206963.html.

4. Richard John Neuhaus, *The End Of Democracy? The Judicial Usurpation of Politics*, ed., Mitchell S. Muncy, (Dallas: Spence Pub. Co., 1997).

5. *Modern Sex: Liberation and Its Discontents*, ed., Myron Magnet, (Chicago: Ivan R Dee, 2001). Lara Riscol, "Bring on the Culture War," (AlterNet: July 22, 2003), http://www.alternet.org/story.html?StoryID=16455.

6. Kreeft's theological approach, while fully orthodox and Catholic, is enriched by the keen attention he gives to the work of non-Catholics such as Martin Luther, C.S. Lewis, and Chuck Colson.

7. Peter Kreeft, *How to Win the Culture War: A Christian Battle Plan for a Society in Crisis*, (Downers Grove, Illinois: InterVarsity Press, 2002), p. 27–30.

8. Ibid., 30–31, 100–106.

9. Ibid., 43.

10. Ibid., 29, 45.

11. Ibid., 39 & 72, 63, 67, 68, 74–79.

12. Ibid., 95. I should note that, in this text, Kreeft does not address or connect the issue of euthanasia to his argument. It would not, however, take much to do so. It follows from Kreeft's argument that the loss of respect for human life originally engender by sexual licentious would expand to encompass the killing of the old and the sick.

13. Ronald Dworkin, *Life's Dominion*, (New York: Vintage Books, 1993).

14. Ibid., 100–101.

15. *Roe v. Wade*, 410 U.S. 133 (1973).

16. *Planned Parenthood of Southeastern Pa. v. Casey*, 505 U.S. 833 (1992).

17. Dworkin, 14.

18. Ibid., 38–39,67.

19. Ibid., 67.

20. Ibid., 100–101.

21. Ibid., x.

22. Fyodor Dostoevsky, *Crime and Punishment*, (New York: Bantam, 1981), 426.

23. Walker Percy, *The Thanatos Syndrome* (New York: Farrar, Strauss, Giroux, 1987), 128.

24. For statistics on the number of abortions performed annually, see, National Right to Life Committee, "Abortion in the United States, Statistics and Trends," http://www.nrlc.org/abortion/facts/abortionstats.html

25. The pro-choice Alan Guttmacher Institute cites 25.9% of all pregnancies ending in abortion. http://www.guttmacher.org/pubs/fb_induced_abortion.html. Also see, Henshaw SK, "Unintended pregnancy in the United States," *Family Planning Perspectives*, 1998, 30(1):24–29 & 46.

26. Alan Guttmacher Institute, "Trends in Abortion in the United States, 1973–2000," http://www.guttmacher.org. Also see, Robert Johnston, "Reasons for Having Abortions in the United States," updated, June 17, 2003. http://www.johnstonarchive.net/policy/abortion/abreason.html.

27. One might object that choosing abortion always results in greater suffering than carrying a child to term as, eventually, the gravity of having killed one's own child begins to sink it and weights on one's conscience. The pro-life movement is right to emphasize that women are also victims of abortion and that from it they suffer irreparable emotional and psychological harm. The ability to experience that harm and, even more so, the ability to anticipate the suffering that will result from having an abortion, is dependent on the woman's psychological and spiritual maturity.

28. The facts recited in this paragraph are drawn from the various articles cited in this section.

29. "A Private Matter," *The Unofficial William H. Macy Site*, http://www2.powercom.net/~brashier/whmacy.

30. *Pro-Life Encyclopedia*, "A Recent History of Abortion in America," American Life League, http://www.eaglecross.net/AborHis.html.

31. Ibid.

32. Edward P. Lazarus, *Closed Chambers*, (New York: Random House, 1998), p. 344.

33. Planned Parenthood Federation of America, Inc., "Family Planning in America," PPFA Web Site, 1998, http://www.plannedparenthood.org/ABOUT/NARRHISTORY/fpam-60.html.

34. Ibid., Alan Guttmacher Institute.

35. For a detailed and insightful critique of this portion of Dworkin's book, and the work as a whole, see Gerard V. Bradley, "Life's Dominion: A Review Essay," *Notre Dame Law Review*, 69:2 (1993): 380–385.

36. Dworkin, 13–14.

37. Ibid., 20.

38. Ibid., 13–14, 20–21.

39. Ibid., 14–15.20–22.

40. The National Right to Life Committee, "The Pro-Life Majorities," http://www.nrlc.org/abortion/major.html. The study cited yielded the following results: "Believe abortion should be prohibited in all circumstances (9%), legal only to save the mother's life (11%), or legal only in the cases of rape, incest or to save the mother's life (33%). (27%) believe abortion should be legal for any reason, but not after the first three months of pregnancy; (5%) believe it should be legal, but not after the first six months; and only (9%) believe abortion should be legal at any time during pregnancy for any reason. *Wirthlin*, November 1994." Thus, the aggregate percentage of the population who believe that abortion should be allowed in cases of rape, incest or maternal life, at least during the first trimester, is 74%. *Wirthlin Worldwide* gathered a slightly different set of survey data in a more recent poll, see http://www.prolifeinfo.org/up16.html.

41. Don Feder, "My Body, My Pellet Gun Defies Logic," *Providence Visitor*, date unknown.

42. "Teen gets 1 1/2 years in baby's death," *Newport Daily News*, July 15, 1997.

43. "Guilty Plea in Baby Death at Prom," *The New York Times on the Web*, http://partners.nytimes.com/aponline/a/AP-Prom-Birth.html?RefId= OpjxYEutt2n2FnKZ.

44. Ibid.

45. "Philadelphia Women Pleads Guilty to Killing Her Eight Children," Associated Press, as reported by Fox News, June 28, 1999, at http://www.foxnews.com/national/062899/infantdeaths.sml.

46. The fact that much suffering comes about as a direct result of a person's own sinful acts is, however politically incorrect, a fundamental truth. This truth, however, should never be an excuse for callousness by Christians towards those in suffering. In no way does the intermediate cause (the ultimate cause of all suffering is original sin) of suffering mitigate our moral obligation to act to relieve our neighbor's suffering. On the self-infliction of most human suffering see, Alice von Hildebrand, "Christianity and the Mystery of Suffering," *The Mind and Heart of the Church*, (San Francisco: Ignatius Press, 1992).

47. See, Martha Beck, *Expecting Adam*, (New York: Times Books/Random House, 1999) and Mary Craig, *Blessings*, (London: Hodder & Stoughton, 1997).

48. Of course, the spiritual and psychological pain caused by "solving" this problem or seeking to escape this suffering by recourse to abortion is incomparably greater.

49. "Atlanta Killer Sought Revenge on the 'Greedy,'" *The Globe and Mail* (Canadian National Edition), Saturday, July 31, 1999.

50. Flannery O'Connor, "Mystery and Manners," *A Memoir of Mary Ann*, The Dominican Nuns of Our Lady of Perpetual Help Home, (New York: Farrar, 1961).

51. "Assisted Suicide Numbers Continue to Rise in Oregon," *American Medical News*, http://www.ama-assn.org/sci-pubs/amnews/pick_03/prsc0324.htm.

52. *Fifth Annual Report on Oregon's Death with Dignity Act*, State of Oregon, Organ Department of Human Services, Health Division, released March 5, 2003. A copy of the full report can be found at www.ohd.hr.state.or.us/cdpe/chs/pas/pas.htm.

53. Ibid. and also see, http://www.ohd.hr.state.or.us/chs/pas/ar-tbl-3.cfm.

54. In at least six states, including Oregon, it is not a crime to assist another person in committing suicide. However, thus far only Oregon funds suicide as part of its Medicaid program. See www.euthanasia.com/bystate.html.

55. A copy of the full list can be downloaded from http://www.ohppr.state.or.us/hsc/PListUpdates/PList-Oct1–2003.pdf.

56. See "Death Stamps: No Joke: Oregon will pay you to die," *Slate,* Miscellaneous Articles, June 2, 1999, www.slate.com/Features/oregon/oregon.asp.

57. David Reinhard, "Liar, Liar" *Sunday Oregonian,* October 19, 1997, editorial page. Reprinted by the International Anti-Euthanasia Task Force, www.iaetf.org/liar.htm.

58. Germain Grisez, "Bioethics and Christian Anthropology," *The National Catholic Bioethics Quarterly* (Vol.1, No.1, Spring 2001)., 34.

59. John Paul II, *Salvifici Doloris,* (Boston: St. Paul Editions, 1984).

60. Plantinga, Alvin, "Philosophers Respond to Pope John Paul II's Encyclical Letter, *Fides et Ratio,*" *Books & Culture,* (Vol. 5: No. 4, July/August 1999).

61. C. S. Lewis, *The Problem of Pain,* (New York: Macmillan, 1962).

62. Ibid., 15.

63. Alice von Hildebrand, "Christianity and the Mystery of Suffering," *The Mind and Heart of the Church,* (San Francisco: Ignatius Press, 1992), p.108.

64. This section of the paper in particular is indebted to a conversation with Germain Grisez and an unpublished paper entitled "The Encounter with Suffering in the Practice of Medicine in the Light of Christian Revelation," forwarded to me by Fr. David Albert Jones, OP.

65. St. Thomas Aquinas, *Summa Theologica,* I-II, q.39, a.4 (Westminster, Maryland: Christian Classics, 1981), 758.

66. The Pope continues "Christ does not explain in the abstract the reasons for suffering, but before all else He says: "Follow me!" Come! Take part through your suffering in this work of saving the world, a salvation achieved through my suffering! Through my cross! Gradually, as the individual takes up His cross, spiritually uniting himself to the cross of Christ, the salvific meaning of suffering is revealed before him." (§26)

2

What is Health? What is Disease?

Jean Bethke Elshtain

In December of 2002, I was invited to deliver a sermon to the adult education class at the St. Charles Baptist Church in New Orleans. This is an old and venerable church that has played an important role in the history of that great city. On that occasion, I talked about the question of abundance, and whether we have lost the concept of what counts as "enough." Let me share with you a bit of what I said on that occasion, for it will lead us into our topic, one that requires that we make certain distinctions we are perhaps unused to making because we have, slothfully—it's always good to pull one of the seven deadly sins into the discussion if you can—acquiesced in certain cultural assumptions that should be challenged, particularly by Christians.

The Lord came that we might have life and have it more abundantly. But, having more abundantly is not the same as the notion that we must have more; that we must acquire more. In our modern culture, we strive, like Fitzgerald's Jay Gatsby, but never quite arrive at the green light beckoning at the end of Daisy's dock. We have lost a concept of enough. By contrast, having life more abundantly relies on our capacity to ask questions about goods and "the good" and to reflect on what we in fact lose in our quest for more. The initial point I am putting into play here is that there are vital distinctions we no longer make between abundance and excess in the material sense. Caught up in the latter we may well abandon, or lose, the former. And we do so at our own peril.

LOSING CRITICAL DISTINCTIONS

Let us turn to health and disease. We all want good health. It is one of life's great blessings. We all fear disease, especially certain diseases: the dread

23

word "cancer," for example. When I was a child one of the dreaded words was "polio" or "infantile paralysis." Those words became a reality for my family and me. The reality was every bit as dreadful as the word. Unsurprisingly, we rejoiced when the polio vaccine came into use. Children now would be spared. Health would triumph over disease. Throughout my lifetime, medical treatments have continued their unprecedented advance.

We have come so far and done so much that even our language has come to reflect this progress. How many times have we heard the word "conquer" when speaking of disease? We speak of a "war" against cancer, the "conquest" of germs, or the "triumph" of modern medicine. Once we conquered polio, we moved on to conquer something else. We are distressed if the war seems to drag on against a disease like cancer. So, we issue reports from the battle-front on a regular basis to see how close we are to a final victory.

Please do not misunderstand me. Making scientific headway against illnesses that lead to terrible human suffering is a great achievement. God gave us minds and the free will to use them properly. Alas, our wills turned against God in that fateful moment in the Garden, so Holy Scripture tells us, and we fell. Forever after, our wills have been flawed; our minds mired in imperfection.

Why mention the "fall" in the same breath as the greatness and inescapability of medical and scientific advance? I do so because we forget on a daily basis that we are fallen; indeed, many are now determined to conquer finitude itself. Mortality has become an illness. There is talk of "immortalization," of creating a world in which my DNA/RNA goes on forever, as if that means that "I" do and death is no more.

When I suggested to a genetics enthusiast that the quest for "immortalization" in the name of health and wellness did not comport with Christian belief, he was genuinely puzzled. When the Lord told us that He came so that we might have life and have it more abundantly, did that not mean that we should devise a way to live forever and in perfect health too? At a wellness clinic I attended, one speaker lectured about the new ideal of human life in the wellness movement. It holds that rather than experiencing any sense of the decline of our powers, we now aspire to stay completely "fit", hale, and hearty, until the day we die. We should not burden ourselves and others up to that point; we should not linger in an unseemly fashion, caught in illness, decrepitude, and dependency. From this perspective, "weakness" is a horror; "helplessness" is the ultimate affront to our dignity.

As in the scenarios of excess, the new concepts of health assume that we cannot have enough. We can always grow fitter—and we should. Only moral slackers devote themselves to other things when, with their spare time, they could be lifting weights, running, or doing aerobic dance. A form of moral censure descends on those who are unfit, unhealthy, and unwell. They likely brought it on themselves and they should shape up immediately! Again, don't get me wrong. As God's creatures we are obliged to respect our bodies and to care for them. We should not treat the great gift of life recklessly. We should not harm our bodies needlessly. But, what is at stake here is a *quest for control*. The underlying assumption seems to be that nature set things up rather badly. We are trapped in finitude. We are not only natals; we are mortals. We need to do something about that. But, in the meantime, we must keep as much control as possible.

I have written and spoken previously on the quest for control and the ways in which we are starting to sort people out by genetic criteria. In our demand for bodily perfection—for a standard of health that weeds out the unfit—we are moving into the realm of eugenics. The body we inhabit is imperfect—unhealthy in some fundamental sense, subject to the vagaries of illness and aging. The future perfect body is our own gleaming fabrication. We measure this body against a standard of health and perfection that promises an endless supply of new body parts via stem cell research for example. Some have even suggested that clones, not being fully human, might be kept alive so that their organs may be harvested to replace the worn-out organs of "real" persons.

There is an irony in all of this. Our culture has become more health conscious. But, we also pride ourselves on our enlightened attitude toward "persons with disabilities," or in the correct terminology of the time, "persons who do not measure up to our standard of fitness." We do not want to deny individual rights or equal access. So, even as we zoom along in our quest for perfect health, we make provisions for those who by definition can never attain such a standard. Just how secure is this concern and how sturdy are these provisions?

DISABILITY AND "DISEASE"

Consider the following. I will put it in the form of a strong thesis: our own liberal society cannot sustain equal regard for persons with disabilities over the long run, especially so if these disabilities are "mental." It cannot do this because our governing presuppositions privilege "choice" as the primary good in human life. Celebrating "choice" as the apogee of human aspiration, we now combine choice with modern technologies of reproductive and genetic engineering. These technologies and our dominant philosophy dictate that it would be far better if persons who are incapable of choosing on the liberal model were not to appear among us. We would be better off as a culture if such persons were not born. Our standard of health suggests as much. So, we strive through genetic engineering and abortion to ensure that such persons are not born. Who would want to be born "unfit," we say in effect?

So strong is the prejudice in this direction that we simply assume that hypothetical unborn children with disabilities would, if they could, choose not to be born. For who would choose to be born with a limitation? Within our dominant framework, persons with handicaps who are among us should be given "access"—another of our buzz words—and they should not be discriminated against unjustly. We have moved beyond the years of hiding people away. But, the fact that such human beings have rights when they live in our midst, does nothing to mitigate new cultural norms that measure progress by a decrease in the number of disabled births.

Despite our modern obsession with diversity, if the "different" stand before us in broken bodies and with broken minds, that is a difference our standard of wellness tells us we should do something to eliminate. The medical profession and the wider culture currently urge the aborting of such human beings. In our brave new world in which all must be born with better health, this admittedly clumsy method can be replaced by a system of "positive" eugenics, as it is called.

One leading bioethicist describes the profoundly retarded and the comatose as "human nonpersons", beings with membership in the human species but with no standing in "the secular moral community."[1] Our modern standard of health supports this arbitrary distinction. Surely, if this attitude comes to prevail on a general scale, the barriers to the elimination of such persons must inexorably wither away. If we follow Holland's lead and approve physician-assisted suicide or medicalized euthanasia, such "human nonpersons" could be eliminated even after birth, as they are now eliminated before birth via selective abortion.

To be sure, many of those who say that the radically "unwell" lack full moral standing do not necessarily think it is a good idea to deprive them of life. Given our religious traditions, public barriers to the killing of persons with severe disabilities remain. But, such barriers are under continuous pressure to succumb to the demands of "secular morality" with its increasingly exclusive interpretation of health and personhood.

Standards of health and illness are not just neutral diagnoses of conditions based on objective medical criteria. Such standards take on a potent normative dimension. They shape, perhaps subtly, the contours of our assessment of what is a good life, a healthy life, a life worth living. If we keep moving in our current cultural direction, it seems likely that, over time, the deeply embedded inhibitions and prohibitions of our moral intuition will slowly but surely give way.

As ethicist Hans S. Reinders (among others) has shown, "people with mental disability [I would extend this to cover all marked disabilities, whether of a mental or physical nature] and their families have reasons to be worried about their future in liberal society. The rapid proliferation of genetic testing may have discriminatory effects . . . because it brings the birth of disabled children within the focus of 'reproductive choice', which makes their parents answerable to the charge of 'irresponsible behavior.'"[2] Responding to a column I had written on the theme of cloning and genetic manipulation, the mother of a Down's syndrome child expressed her deep foreboding on this very theme. She worried about societal provision and assistance for persons with disabilities and their families should the time come—and it seems to be approaching rapidly—when parents who chose to bring an unhealthy child into the world would be labeled irresponsible for burdening that child and the society with unnecessary suffering. Why should *we*, the healthy, support those who have chosen irresponsibly in favor of disease, a condition we regard as unhealthy in the deepest, one might even say, ontological sense?

None of what I have been saying is the stuff of science fiction. It is the texture of our ethical lives at this moment. The urgency to eliminate flaws is palpable. Our understanding of humanity narrows as our normative ideal of what counts as a healthy person, free from illness, expands. Accepting the unwell and those with disabilities, becomes for us an ever more arduous task. This leads me to the unhappy conclusion that a liberal culture, a good and brilliant culture in so many ways, is not in a strong position to sustain support for the unwell, particularly if it takes the form of prolonged illness or disability. Our quest for control and prevention pushes us toward the elimination of certain conditions, which at some point in the future may invite the elimination of certain human persons on the grounds that they are not full fledged members of the secular moral community.

TO HEAL AND TO CURE: IS THERE A DIFFERENCE?

Some of you, at this point, may be wondering how all of this pertains to Jesus' healing mission. Did not Jesus eliminate disease? Did He not make the lame walk and the blind see? Was He not, in His own way, working to eliminate flaws and imperfections? I am not a Biblical exegete, nor even a theologian, but putting the questions this way is surely not adequate and misses something basic. For Jesus helps us to think about another critical distinction that we systematically eliminate or elide altogether nowadays. I refer to the distinction between *curing* and *healing*.

Let us remind ourselves of a few of these Scriptural moments, all drawn from the Gospel of Matthew. Matthew 8: 5–17 recounts the story of Jesus healing a paralyzed servant who is in terrible distress. When the centurion in Capernaum tells the Lord of his servant in distress, Jesus says, "I will come and heal him." The centurion tells Jesus that he is unworthy for the Lord to enter under his roof—"only say the word and my servant will be healed." When Jesus hears this humble admission, He remarks "even in Israel . . . I have not found such faith." Jesus then sends the man forth with the words: ". . . be it done for you as you have believed." And, we are told, "the servant was healed at that very moment."

Hard upon this story comes one about Peter's mother-in-law lying sick with fever. Jesus touches her and she is healed. Then, the same evening, many "who were possessed with demons" were brought to Him. Matthew tells us that He cast out the evil spirits "with a word, and healed all who were sick." They are not cured but healed. The healing mission continues with the famous story, in Matthew 9, of the ruler who comes to Jesus, telling Him that his daughter has died. He pleads with Jesus to come with him and to lay His hand on her, for then "she will live."

Following the ruler, Jesus is in turn followed by a woman "who had suffered from a hemorrhage for twelve years. She touches the fringe of Jesus' garment, believing that if she can but touch the garment she will be made well. Jesus turns, sees her, and tells her to take heart "for your faith has made you well." Upon arriving at the ruler's house, Jesus tells the grieving to depart, for the girl is only sleeping. The crowd laughs but the girl rises when Jesus takes her by the hand.

Throughout the district word spreads. Blind men follow Him. It is their expression of belief prior to the Lord's touch that is essential to their healing. Matthew 15 tells another story of demonic possession. We learn of the plea of a Canaanite woman who begs Jesus to have mercy on her, for "my daughter is severely possessed by a demon." The disciples want to send her away. We get the impression that her pleading is a nuisance. Jesus initially says that he has been sent to the lost sheep of Israel, but the woman's faith touches him. "Great is your faith," He proclaims, and her daughter is healed.

What are we to make of all this? Should contemporary Christians be a bit embarrassed because the healing miracles seem rather, well, fantastic? Some even find the healing miracles problematic because, they say, the stories suggest that something is "wrong" with being lame, blind, bleeding profusely, or possessed by a demon (read as mental illness). Nowadays, in the manner that Scripture does, our contemporary prejudices get in the way of our understanding.

These stories help us to reflect on the distinction between a cure in the modern medical sense and healing in the Biblical sense. The removal of bodily symptoms signifies an inward shift—from distress and derangement to healing. Your faith has made you well; has made you whole. Remember that elsewhere Jesus chides those of little faith who require external signs for everything: those who demand evidence—and all of us, at one time or another, are such persons. The key to authentic healing, the stories tell us, is faith. Healing can occur in the absence of a cure and that is precisely the distinction that our modern culture does not understand.

I witnessed this kind of healing years ago as a polio patient at the Children's Hospital in Denver, Colorado. Some children were healed without being cured, while others, who were sometimes better off than many of the rest of us, were neither healed nor cured. These children often grew silent and depressed. They became angry and anxious. Others approached their illness with sadness, but also with calm and determination. What made the difference?

Obviously, I cannot explore this question as an empirical matter. But, I can affirm that in the absence of a cure there can be healing. It is the recognition of this most important truth that we are in danger of losing. We act as if the absence of a cure is a violent affront to human life. Studies of the stories of dying children suggest that the children who were healed before dying of their illnesses were those whose families were able to let go of anger and find meaning in their suffering. The children who were neither cured nor healed were ill-served by frightened parents and frustrated doctors who considered childhood illness a meaningless evil. Parents and doctors who were angry and frightened themselves considered health to be the highest good. Consumed by an obsession with health, they could not look beyond illness and disability. Today, there is a powerful need for healing, but in our monomaniacal search for a cure; healing eludes us.

In 1944, C.S. Lewis published a prescient book called, *The Abolition of Man*.[3] Lewis lamented certain developments in education that focused more on our own subjective sentiments than on authentic human value and on the human engagement with the world. The approach he criticized was incurably present-minded, believing that the past was fit only for overcoming. As a result, we lose the strength of tradition and move into a world of "false" by contrast to "just" sentiments. We will pay a heavy price for this dereliction, Lewis predicted, for "a famished nature will be avenged and a hard heart is no infallible protection against a soft head."[4]

Lewis argued that the abolition of man was our alleged "conquest of nature." He worried about "selective breeding" and the terrible implications of eugenics. He worried about the pretension that applied psychology would lead us to believe we had full control over ourselves and the satiation of all our needs. That seems far more manageable than seeking what is good. We would no longer be able to distinguish what is "corrupt" and "degenerate" because these "imply a doctrine of value" and any such doctrine is meaningless.[5]

Our inability to distinguish healing from cure; our refusal to reflect critically on the exponential leap in our standards of what counts as health or wellness and the dark underside of these developments—all attest to the prior 'abolition of man' of which Lewis writes. That lurks throughout my discussion. What is our understanding of the dignity of the human person? In what does this dignity consist? Who is and who is not within the boundary of full moral concern? Inevitably, questions of health and disease lead us back to these first order questions. And that is as it should be.

NOTES

1. The quotes are from Tristam Engelhardt as cited by Hans S. Reinders in his book, *The Future of The Disabled in Liberal Society: An Ethical Analysis* (Notre Dame: Notre Dame University Press, 2000), p.108.

2. Reinders, *Ibid.*, p. x.

3. San Francisco: Zondervan Publishing House, HarperSanFrancisco, 1974.

4. *Ibid.*, p. 14.

5. *Ibid.*, p. 65.

II

PHILOSOPHICAL ROOTS OF THE MORAL DEBATE

3

Are There Specific Exceptionless Moral Norms?

Patrick Lee

Let me begin with a specific example. In his book *Situation Ethics,* Joseph Fletcher tells the story of Mrs. Bergmeier. She was a German housewife who was imprisoned by the Russians in the Ukraine during World War II, and thus separated from her family in Germany. Mrs. Bergmeier discovered that she could be reunited with her family if she were pregnant. Pregnant prisoners were considered by the Russians to be a liability. So Mrs. Bergmeier asked a camp guard to impregnate her, which he was happy to do. When she became pregnant she was released from the camp and returned to Germany and her family.

Joseph Fletcher praised Mrs. Bergmeir's action for demonstrating that we should not be bound by absolute rules and regulations, but should wait for the particular situation to see what the loving thing to do is. The question about this situation would be: is adultery *always* morally wrong, or are there some situations, perhaps very few, in which it is the right thing, the loving thing, to do?

Some people argue that there is not any specific type of action that you can say is always morally wrong. This would mean that you cannot say that adultery is always morally wrong, nor intentionally killing innocent people, nor euthanasia, abortion, sterilization, premarital sex, and so on. Of course, these people might grant that such acts are *usually* or *in general* morally wrong, but you cannot say, according to some, that any of these specific types of acts is always morally wrong.

Allow me to say a bit more about this question before I examine the arguments for and against. The question is: are there *specific* exceptionless moral norms? Almost everyone admits that there are *general* principles which are true without exception (act out of love, act justly, and so on).

There is a fierce debate, however, about whether there are any *specific* exceptionless moral norms, that is, moral norms that exclude specific types of choices. Is there any specific type of act or specific type of choice that we ought to never do, no matter what the circumstances and no matter what consequences we expect to follow from them?

On this issue, there *is* a great deal of debate. This is, I would venture to say, one of those key questions in what is often called a culture war—some people want to take the culture one way and others want to take it the other way. I am going to argue that there *are* specific exceptionless moral norms and that they are important to the moral life because they help define our attitude to the intrinsic goods of persons.

So, why would someone say the opposite—why would someone say that there are no specific exceptionless moral norms? There are, I think, basically two approaches or two types of defense for this position: one is *situation ethics (situationism)*, and the other is called *consequentialism* (sometimes: *utilitarianism or proportionalism*). In this paper, I will do four things. First, reply to situationism, second, reply to utilitarianism, third, set out some of the positive reasons for the position that there are specific exceptionless moral norms, and fourth, reply to two common objections to this position. I will set out the positive reasons for the position (that there are exceptionless moral norms), while answering the opposed positions.

ON SITUATIONISM OR PARTICULARISM

Situationism claims that we cannot know in advance what the right thing to do will be in a specific situation. There may be something unique in a particular situation that tells us to throw out the general rules. So, the situationist, in effect, says that we know what is right or wrong by an intuition into the particular situation. And so, according to them, there are no moral absolutes. This position is also sometimes called *"particularism."*

There are various difficulties with particularism. For one thing, it wipes out the unity of the moral life. From the particularist point-of-view, what I do tomorrow may have very little to do with what I do today. My life becomes just a series of morally unrelated episodes, similar to a Seinfeld TV show.

An even more serious difficulty is that, in the concrete, it is difficult to tell the difference between having an intuition and just having a strong, but misguided, emotion. In other words, in the concrete this theory is simply unworkable. For example: a young couple kissing in the back seat of a car at the end of their date have an "intuition" that premarital sex is not always wrong—but was it really an intuition or was it a very strong feeling? The same thing could happen in a euthanasia case: a person is in extreme pain and there is virtually no hope of being cured. He seems to have an intuition that euthanasia in this case is the morally right thing to do. But, was it really an intuition or was it just a strong feeling?

The central difficulty is as follows. There are intelligible features of moral actions that are repeatable, or able to be instantiated in several instances. And there are some intelligible features of moral actions that violate the basic and most general moral norm. Of course, this supposes a position based on at least some general moral criteria. However, there are human actions with certain features that will always be morally wrong, whether, for example, one is a natural law theorist or a Kantian ethical theorist. Since I am a natural law ethical theorist, I will try to explain the basis of moral absolutes from that standpoint.

Here is how I would explain that basis. There are various basic, intrinsic goods of human persons. For example, life, health, knowledge of truth, friendship, self-integration, and so on—these are intrinsic perfections of human persons. And the basic moral criterion is this: we should respect all of these basic goods, both in ourselves and in others, in all of our actions.

The basic idea is that whenever we choose; we choose to pursue one or more of these basic goods—or at least some aspect of a basic good—in some way or another. The moral norm is *not* that we should pursue all of the basic goods all of the time—that is not possible. When we choose, we are choosing to pursue one basic good and thus not pursuing many other goods at the same time. But, we can have two different attitudes toward those other goods not chosen. First, we can choose to pursue one good rather than others, but in such a way as to remain open and respectful to the basic goods not chosen. That is a morally good choice. On the other hand, it is also true that we often choose to pursue one instance of a basic good (or just an aspect of a basic good, such as pleasure), but in such a way as to denigrate another instance (or instances) of a basic human good. That is, we often choose to pursue a good, but in such a way as to suppress or unduly neglect —in other words treat as a non-good—another instance of a basic human good.[1]

For example, consider a hit-man, someone who takes pay to kill others. He may be doing this to support himself and his family, thus pursuing a good, but he is doing so by means of suppressing other instances of basic goods, namely human lives. In the Mrs. Bergmeier case, she is pursuing the basic goods of life and family, but her choice violates the good of marriage, and also the personal integrity of the prison guard who "helps" her. In such acts, by the very nature of these choices, one suppresses one's appreciation for a basic human good. So, we can say in contrast to situationism or particularism that there are certain types of choices which by their very nature involve a *closing of one's will to one or more of the basic human goods*, and for that reason are wrong no matter what the circumstances and no matter what the consequences we expect will follow.

CONSEQUENTIALISM OR UTILITARIANISM

A second reason why someone might deny that there are moral absolutes is certainly more popular. This is the utilitarian position. According to utilitarianism, sometimes it is morally right to destroy, damage, or impede one instance of a basic good in order to bring about a greater good in the long-run, or perhaps, the least bad consequences in the long-run.

The Mrs. Bergmeier case seems to be an example where someone would argue in this way. Why would someone say that Mrs. Bergmeier's act was the morally right thing to do? (Please note that we are discussing the *objective* morality of acts, not the guilt or innocence of those who perform that act or choice: someone may act from an erroneous conscience, and if he is not at fault for his error in conscience—an important if—then he is not at fault for his act). They might say it is okay because it produces the best consequences in the long-run or at least avoided very bad consequences.

Or again, consider the issue of cloning or using human embryos for stem cell research. Why would someone justify this? One might argue that destroying nascent human life is justified because of the great good that might come from it—the curing of various diseases such as Parkinson's or spinal chord injuries. So, from this point-of-view, there are no moral absolutes— that is, no specific exceptionless moral norms—because there could, in principle, always arise some situation in which doing the type of act you are talking about would appear to produce the best consequences in the long-run or the least bad consequences in the long run. That is, it may be necessary according to utilitarianism—that is, morally right—to do evil (not *moral* evil, but the destruction, damaging or impeding of a basic good) so that good may come from it. So, this would apply to *any* type of act: intentionally killing an innocent person, adultery, rape, torture, and so on. There is no type of act that could not, on this view, be the morally right thing to do in certain circumstances.

I will present two arguments against this theory. First, I think there is an indication that something is wrong with this theory because if it were really adopted, it would change how we are *now* related to every other human person, including especially those we are close to. Suppose I could save five people from certain death by torturing or killing one of my children. Would it be right for me to act against one intrinsic good of a person (my child's life or health) in order to prevent these very bad consequences?

A utilitarian or consequentialist might agree that this would not be right. They might say that the impact on my relationship to my child is an important consequence that outweighs the other consequences. But this suggests the question: Suppose I could save six, or seven, or—and keep adding to the number. Is there a point at which I should torture or kill my own child? *And the point of my questions here is this: It seems that any readiness on my part to kill my child for the sake of some overall net benefit would utterly change the attitude I have now toward that child.* The same point could be made about torture: a readiness to torture my child if necessary to avoid terrible consequences would change my relationship to him. Instead of having an unconditional love for him, I would be viewing his welfare, his life, as something to be cherished *only if* it fits in with the well-being of the whole, the group. In that case, my love for the whole might seem to be unconditional, but I would be ready to exclude my child from my concern, since I would be ready to will his destruction as a means of preventing harm to the whole. But such readiness, I submit, is contrary to the love and respect that we are called to have—not only for our children, though especially and foremost for them, but for every person. We should exclude *no* person from the circle of those for whom we care about for their own sake, regardless of whether, "the greatest good for the greatest number" or "the best consequences in the long-run," are served well or ill. Utilitarianism or consequentialism makes each individual life and each aspect of each individual—his health, his knowledge of truth, his friendships, his marriage, and so on—dispensable in relation to a larger group or whole.

Moral actions are not just physical behaviors that last but a short time. Rather, the physical behavior is morally significant insofar as it carries out a choice or act of will. In choosing, one disposes oneself in this direction or that direction. While the behavior may be transitory, this shaping of oneself remains as an aspect of oneself, unless one later repents. So, if one chooses contrary to a basic human good (that is, contrary to an intrinsic aspect of a human person), one disposes oneself against that good. Such choices diminish or suppress in oneself an appreciation for some aspect of the intrinsic good of real human persons. And so, there are certain types of acts that are always wrong because they necessarily involve a suppression of respect for an intrinsic basic good of a human person.

There is a second problem—equally serious—with the utilitarian or consequentialist position. The second problem has to do with what it means to speak about "best consequences in the long run" or the "greatest net good." Let's look again at what the utilitarian or consequentialist is saying. He posits: It is okay to destroy, damage, or impede one instance of a basic good in order to avoid very bad consequences in the long run. In other words, what he is saying is that I get into a situation in which I can see that doing X—say intentionally killing someone or sterilizing myself or my wife—would bring about an overall lesser evil than if I do the opposite. So, the consequentialist is saying that I have a choice between action A and action B, and I can see that the consequences of B will be much worse than the consequences of A. And, that is why it is morally right, according to him, to act directly against a basic good, such as life, knowledge of truth, marriage, or so on. But, this will only work if I can do the following:

1. I have to be able to figure out what the consequences of A will be and what the consequences of B will be—at least in a rough way.
2. I have to be able to measure the net goodness or badness of the consequences of A in relation to the net goodness or badness of the consequences of B.

In order to make this second judgment I have to be able to say: the future state of the world will be overall better off if I do A than if I do B. But am I really in a position to make such a judgment? Is that kind of judgment even possible in a situation in which I have free choice?

To see that it is not possible, and also to see in more detail what is fundamentally wrong with utilitarianism and consequentialism, we need to look more closely at situations in which we have a moral choice, situations where there is a moral option.

There is a moral option, a moral issue, only in situations where we really have a free choice—where we could do A or we could do B, or at least where we could do A or not do A. If we are determined by our antecedent conditions, then we really do not have a free choice, and we really do not have a moral option. If we do not have a free choice, then we are just doing what we are determined to do, and we are neither to be praised nor blamed for our actions.

But, suppose I could do what the utilitarian claims that I must do in order to figure out what the right thing to do is. Suppose I *could* tally up what the consequences of A and B will be and then measure them against one another. So, suppose I conclude that A will result in 30 units of bad but B will result in 40 units of bad. Well, in that situation, do I really have a free choice? If I can really say that option A will produce 30 units of bad, but B will produce 40 units of bad, then how *could* I choose B. The answer, I think, is that I could not. If option B is simply speaking worse than option A, that is, if it is worse in every respect than option A, then there could be *no point* to choosing option B. So, I have a free choice only if I see something good in one alternative and a different kind of good in another alternative (even if the "good" is an avoiding of a distinctive bad). In order to have free choice, the goodness (or badness) in the options for choice must be *incommensurable*. In other words, whenever the utilitarian calculus can be applied, then I have no free choice. But, the point of a moral theory is to provide guidance for free choices. So, the utilitarian theory simply does not offer me guidance for any situation in which a moral choice has to be made.

This is not just a debater's point against utilitarianism. The point is that whenever I have a free choice, I am faced with a situation in which the goods and bads in one option are incommensurable with the goods and bads of the other option. And, this is because we are talking about different instances of intrinsic goods, and my attitudes—my openness to or being closed to—each of these intrinsic goods. But, to make a utilitarian choice is to take the attitude that these really *are not* irreducibly distinctive types of intrinsic goods, but rather are just so many quantities of good that can be measured against one another. It is, in other words, to adopt the attitude that the goods I act against—such goods as life, health, knowledge of truth, and marriage—are really only measurable *and therefore instrumental goods*. It is to demote these goods to a lower level, to adopt the attitude that they really *are not* intrinsically good. And so, to act on the utilitarian principle is to take on the attitude that the basic good deliberately destroyed (or damaged or impeded) is quantifiably lesser than the goods chosen, and that means I am taking the attitude that the unchosen good is not really an *irreducibly basic human good.*

Now, there are several objections that could be raised to this position, but I would like to consider briefly two objections that are commonly raised.

First, one might object as follows: I have maintained that one should not do evil that good may come from it. That one ought to never act directly against a basic human good or unduly neglect a basic good. But, it might be objected, sometimes we get into a situation in which whatever we do, we are going to cause a great evil, a death, sterility, a loss of trust, or so on. Isn't it the case, the objection might be raised, that in some situations *both* options are evil, and so we cannot say that we ought to never do evil?

To reply: it is important to distinguish between directly willing something and intending it, as opposed to causing it as a side effect. For example, there is a significant difference between choosing to kill as a means toward some good end versus choosing to do something that has, as a *side effect*, the destruction or damaging of some basic human good.

For example, there is a difference between choosing to kill someone as a means toward ending his suffering or as a means toward not-being-responsible for a child—which I maintain is always objectively morally wrong—and someone with cancer choosing not take a course of chemo-therapy even though it may bring about an early death as a side effect. Or again, direct killing, that is, choosing death as a means, is different from what occurs, say, when a pregnant woman has an aggressive cancer in her uterus. It is permissible in that case to remove the uterus with the unborn child inside. This will cause the baby's death, but it is neither an end nor a means; rather, it is a side effect of removing the cancerous uterus.

So, let us return to the objection. In some cases, whatever we do we will cause some evil. My answer is that, yes, there are such cases—that is, cases where whatever we do some evil (a non-moral evil) will result. But, there are never any cases where we cannot avoid *choosing* the destruction, damaging, or impeding of a basic human good.

Such destruction or diminishing of basic goods as a side effect of what one does is not the same as choosing against a basic good, and so it does not necessarily involve a lack of appreciation or commitment to those goods that are diminished (or destroyed) as a side effect. Indeed, such diminishing or destruction of basic goods *as a side effect* is strictly unavoidable. Every choice we make is a choice to pursue and enhance some goods and not others. Thus, every choice we make involves a non-realization and thus a diminishing of other basic goods.

On the other hand, a choice to act directly against a basic human good *is* incompatible with an appreciation and respect for the intrinsic goods of persons. Such a choice involves, at least implicitly, the judgment that some basic goods of persons, some intrinsic aspects of persons, are not inherently worthwhile, but are worthwhile only if they fit into one's moral calculus.

It has sometimes been objected that there really is no morally significant difference between directly doing evil and causing evil as a side effect.[2] Therefore, (the argument continues) since everyone admits that it is sometimes morally right to cause evil as a side effect, then it is also, in some cases, morally right to act directly against a basic human good. However, this argument is surely mistaken. If, for example, killing were the same as causing death as a side effect, then *everything* we did other than life-saving attempts would be cases of killing. Thus, in every choice we make to pursue some good other than the saving of someone's life, we are doing something which has the side effect of *not* saving someone's life. If this objection were correct, then the choice to take one's children for a walk rather than saving the street children of Calcutta would be as murderous as deliberately blanketing those same children with machine gun bullets.[3] We cannot pursue all of the basic goods all of the time, but we can and ought to refrain from directly willing to destroy, damage, or impede a basic human good.

A second objection to the existence of moral absolutes (specific exceptionless moral norms) might be expressed as follows:

"Aren't you in the end just giving priority to abstract rules instead real, concrete people? The basic general norm should be love—love one another. But sometimes love requires us to do evil, or to do a little evil, in order to protect or respect real live people. Aren't you engaging in a kind of rule worship? We should care more about helping real people. And sometimes that means saying to hell with your rules, let's help these real people in front of us."

This is a very common notion of morality, and in particular it is a common misconception of what natural law theory is all about. So, I think it is important to reply to it. The answer is that the basic moral criterion is not a set of abstract rules. Nor is it an abstract nature, an abstract pattern as it were, discerned in our natures. Rather, the basic moral norm is really the various basic human goods to which we are naturally inclined. And these are the intrinsic aspects of real human persons—they are not abstractions at all. So, to act contrary to an absolute moral norm is not to violate some arbitrary rule. Rather, it is to turn one's will against the intrinsic aspect, an intrinsic good, of a real human person.

We could also put the point this way. The objection was that sometimes we should throw away the rules and just follow love. Well, that cannot apply to the basic moral principles, which I have been speaking about. To love someone is to will to them what is genuinely good. For example, to love my children is to will to them that they be healthy, morally upright, knowledgeable, etc. So, to love persons involves willing their real fulfillment. But, their real fulfillment is just the various basic human goods we have spoken about here. So, the basic moral criterion is really just articulating what is specifically required by a consistent love of persons. It makes no sense to say that I am going to set aside the rules and love you, if loving you involves acting directly against some intrinsic good of you or someone else.

In sum, I have set out a positive case for exceptionless moral norms. There are various basic human goods, the perfections of human persons as human persons. We should energetically pursue some of these (we cannot pursue all of them all of the time) for ourselves and others, and we ought to never act directly against any of them. I argued against situationism: there *are* repeatable features of acts which render any acts of certain sorts objectively morally wrong, no matter what the circumstances. I replied to utilitarianism or consequentialism, which reduces each individual good to something entirely dispensable in relation to a collective state of affairs (the best consequences in the long-run or the greatest good). It requires that we attempt to measure against one another what cannot in truth be measured. Finally, we examined two common objections to specific exceptionless moral norms and found them to be grounded in confusions about the basis of moral goodness. St. Paul was, of course, right: we ought to never do evil that good may come from it (Rm. 3: 8).

NOTES

1. For the approach taken here, see Germain Grisez and Russell Shaw, *Beyond the New Morality, the Responsibilities of Freedom, 3rd ed.* (Notre Dame, Ind.: University of Notre Dame Press, 1988).

2. For example, James Rachels, "Active and Passive Euthanasia," reprinted in several places, for example: *Social Ethics, Morality and Social Policy, 5th ed.*, ed. Thomas A. Mappes and Jane S. Zembaty (New York: McGraw-Hill, 1997), 61–66.

3. John Finnis, "Understanding the Case Against Euthanasia," in *Euthanasia Examined, Ethical, Legal and Clinical Perspectives*, ed. John Keown (New York: Cambridge University Press, 1995), 64–65.

4

A Refutation of Moral Relativism

Peter Kreeft

PURPOSE

Peter Maurin and Dorothy Day defined a good society as one that made it easy to be good. Correlatively, a free society is one that makes it easy to be free.

To be free, and to live freely, is to live spiritually. Only spirit, not matter, is free. To live spiritually is to live morally. The two essential powers of spirit that distinguish it from matter are intellect and will, the capacity for knowledge and moral choice, awareness of truth and goodness.

The most radical threat to living morally today is the loss of moral principles. Moral practice has always been difficult for fallen humanity, but at least there has always been the lighthouse of moral principles, no matter how stormy the sea of moral practice may have become. Today, for the majority of our mind-molders, in formal education or informal education (i.e. media), the light is gone. Morality is a fog of feelings. That is why to them, as Chesterton said, morality is always dreadfully complicated—to a man who has lost his principles.

Principles mean moral absolutes, unchanging rocks beneath the changing waves of feelings and practice. Moral relativism is the philosophy that denies moral absolutes. That philosophy is the Prime Suspect, Public Enemy Number One. That is the philosophy that has extinguished the light in the minds of our teachers, and then our students, and eventually, if not reversed, will extinguish our whole civilization.

Therefore, I do not want to just present a good case against moral relativism, but to refute it, to unmask it, to strip it naked, to humiliate it, to shame it, to give it the "whoopin" it deserves (as they say in America's good neighbor to the south, Texas).

DEFINITIONS

We must begin with a definition. Moral relativism usually includes three claims: that morality is (1) changeable, (2) subjective, and (3) individual; that it is relative, first, to changing times ("You can't turn back the clock"), second, to what we subjectively think or feel ("There is nothing good or bad, but thinking makes it so"), and third, to different individuals or groups ("Different strokes for different folks"). Moral absolutism claims that there are moral principles that are (1) unchangeable, (2) objective, and (3) universal.

THE IMPORTANCE OF THE ISSUE

How important is this issue? After all, it's just philosophy, just "ideas." But, ideas have consequences. Sometimes these consequences are as momentous as a Holocaust; sometimes even more momentous.

Philosophy is just thought. But, "sow a thought, reap an act; sow an act, reap a habit; sow a habit, reap a character; sow a character, reap a destiny." That is true for societies just as it is for individuals.

How important is the issue? It is only the single most important issue of our age. No society in history has ever survived without rejecting this philosophy. There has never been a society of moral relativists. Therefore, there are only three possibilities. Our society will either (1) disprove one of the most universally established of all the laws of human history, or (2) repent of its relativism and survive, or (3) persist in its relativism and perish.

How important is the issue? CS. Lewis says, in "The Poison of Subjectivism," that relativism "will certainly end our species and . . . damn our souls." (Please remember that Oxonians are not given to exaggeration.)

Why "damn our souls"? Because Lewis, as a Christian, does not dare to disagree with the fundamental teaching of his Lord (and of all the prophets in His Jewish tradition) that salvation presupposes repentance, and repentance presupposes an objectively real moral law. Moral relativism eliminates that law, trivializes repentance, and imperils salvation.

Why "end our species" and not our modern Western culture? Because the entire human species is becoming increasingly westernized and relativized. The malignant moral cancer is metastasizing. And America is the primary place to stop it because America is the primary site from which it is spreading.

It is ironic that this "primary site" is also the West's most religious nation. It is ironic because religion is to relativism what Dr. Van Helsing is to Count Dracula. Within America, the strongest opposition to relativism is in the churches. But—still further irony—polls show that Catholics are just as relativistic, in both belief and practice, as non-Catholics; that 62% of Evangelicals say they disbelieve in any absolute truths; and American Jews are significantly more relativistic than Gentiles. Only Orthodox Jews, Eastern Orthodox, and Fundamentalists seem to be resisting the culture, but only by withdrawing from it. That includes most Muslims, except for the minority who terrorize it.

When Pat Buchanan told us, at the 1992 Republican convention, that we were in a "culture war," nearly everyone laughed, sneered, or barked at him. Today, nearly everyone knows he was right. And the "culture war" is most centrally about this issue.

THE ARGUMENTS FOR RELATIVISM REFUTED

The arguments for relativism will first be examined and then refuted to clear the way for opposing arguments.

(1) The Argument against Guilt

The first argument is psychological. In practice, psychological "becauses" (i.e. subjective personal motives) are a more powerful source of moral relativism than logical "becauses" (i.e. objective logical arguments). What is the main motive for relativism? Since our deepest desire is for happiness, and since fears correspond to desires, it is probably the fear that absolutism would make us unhappy by making us feel guilty. That is why absolutism is often called "unloving" or "uncompassionate".

Turned into an argument, it looks like this: Good morality has good consequences and bad morality has bad consequences. Feelings of unhappiness and guilt are bad consequences, while feelings of happiness and self-esteem are good consequences. Moral absolutism produces the bad feelings of guilt and unhappiness, while moral relativism produces the good feelings of self-esteem and happiness. Therefore, moral absolutism is bad and moral relativism is good.

Reply

(a) The answer to this argument is, first of all, that absolute moral law exists to maximize happiness, not to minimize it, and therefore it is maximally loving and compassionate—like labels on poison bottles, or fences at the edge of a cliff.

(b) But what about guilt? Removing moral absolutes does indeed remove guilt, and guilt obviously does not make you happy, at least in the short run. But guilt, like physical pain, may be necessary to avoid much greater unhappiness in the long run—if it is realistic, that is, in tune with reality. The question is: Does reality include objective moral laws? If not, guilt is an experience as pointless as paranoia. If so, it is as proper as pain, and it is there for a similar reason: to prevent harm. Guilt is a warning in the soul analogous to pain as a warning in the body.

(c) The relativist's argument also has a question-begging assumption: that feelings are the standard for judging morality. But, the claim of traditional morality is exactly the opposite: that morality is the standard for judging feelings.

(d) Finally, if the argument from guilt vs. self-esteem is correct, the absurd conclusion follows that if rapists, cannibals, terrorists or tyrants feel self-esteem, they are better off than if they feel guilty; that Hitler's problem was not too much self-esteem but too little. Some ideas are beyond the need for refutation except in universities.

(2) The Argument from Cultural Relativity

A second argument for relativism is the argument from cultural relativity. The argument seems impregnable, for the claim is that anthropologists and sociologists have discovered moral relativism to be an empirical fact; that different cultures and societies, like different individuals, do in fact have very different moral values. In Eskimo culture and in Holland, killing old people is right; in America east of Oregon it is wrong. In contemporary culture, fornication is right; in Christian cultures it's wrong. And so forth.

In the *Discourse on Method*, Descartes notes that there is no idea so strange that some philosopher has not seriously taught it. Similarly, there is no practice so strange that some society has not legitimized it (e.g. genocide or cannibalism) or so innocent that some society has not forbidden it (e.g. entering a temple with a hat on, or without one). So, anyone who thinks values are not relative to cultures is simply ignorant of facts.

Reply

(a) To see the logical fallacy in this apparently impregnable argument, we need to look at its unspoken assumption, which is that moral rightness is defined by obedience to cultural values; that it is right to obey your culture's values. Only if we combine that hidden premise with the stated premise, that values differ with different cultures, do we get the conclusion that moral rightness differs with cultures, that what is wrong in one culture is right in another. But, surely this hidden premise begs the question. It presupposes the very moral relativism it is supposed to prove. The absolutist denies that it is always right to obey your culture's values. He has a trans-cultural standard by which he can criticize a whole culture's values; that is why he can be a progressive and a radical, while the relativist can only be a status quo conservative, having no higher standard than his culture. Only massive media "Big Lie" propaganda could have so confused people's minds that they spontaneously think the opposite. In fact, it is only the believer in the old-fashioned Natural Moral Law who can be a moral radical and progressive in his society. He alone can say to a Hitler or a Saddam Hussein, "You and your whole social order are wrong, and wicked, and deserve to be destroyed." The relativist can only say, "Different strokes for different folks, and I happen to like my strokes better than yours, that's all."

(b) A second logical weakness of the argument about cultural relativism is its equivocation on the term "values." The absolutist distinguishes subjective opinions about values from objectively true values just as he distinguishes objective truth from subjective opinions about God, or life after death, or happiness, or numbers, or beauty (just to take five other non-empirical things). It may be difficult, or even impossible, to prove these things, or to attain certainty about them, or even to know them at all; but that does not mean they are unreal. Even if these things cannot be known, it does not follow that they are unreal. Even if they cannot be known with certainty, it does not follow that they cannot be known. (They might be known by "right opinion".) Even if they cannot be proved, it does not follow that they cannot be known with certainty. And even if they cannot be proved by the scientific method, it does not follow that they cannot be proved at all. They could be (1) real even if (2) unknown, (2) known even if not (3) certainly known, (3) certainly known even if not (4) proved, and (4) proved even if not (5) scientifically proved. There are five different questions here, not just one.

The equivocation in the cultural relativist's argument is between value opinions and values. Different cultures may have different opinions about what is morally valuable, just as they may have different opinions about what happens after death. These disagreements, however, do not entail the conclusion that what is right in one culture is wrong in another any more than different opinions about the afterlife entail the conclusion that different things happen after death depending on different cultural opinions (or individual opinions). For example, just because I may believe there is no Hell does not prove there is none, or that I will not go there. Similarly, just because a good Nazi thinks genocide is right does not prove it is right—unless, of course, there is nothing more to right and wrong than thinking that makes it so. But, that is the relativist's conclusion. It cannot also be his premise without begging the question.

(c) There is still another error in the cultural relativist's argument. The argument from "facts" doesn't even have its facts right. Cultures do not in fact differ totally about values, even if the term "values" is taken to mean merely "value opinions". No culture ever existed that believed and taught what Nietzsche called for: a "transvaluation of all values." There have been differences in emphasis—e.g. our ancestors valued courage more and compassion less—but there has never been anything like the relativism of opinions about basic moral values that the relativist teaches as factual history. Just imagine what that would be like. Try to imagine a society where charity, justice, honesty, courage, wisdom, hope, and self-control were deemed morally evil, and unrestricted selfishness, injustice, lying, cowardice, foolishness, despair, and uncontrolled addiction were deemed morally good. Such a society is never found on earth. If it exists anywhere, it is only in Hell (and its colonies). Only Satan and his worshippers say "Evil, be thou my good."

There are important disagreements about values between cultures, but beneath all disagreements about lesser values (e.g. money) lies agreement about more basic ones (e.g. justice). And beneath all disagreement about applying values to situations (e.g. should we have capital punishment?) lies agreement about the values to be applied (e.g. murder is evil, since human life is good). Moral disagreements, between cultures as well as between individuals, would be impossible unless there were some deeper moral agreements, some common moral premises.

Morals are to mores what concepts are to words. When you visit a foreign country the language seems totally different at first. But, then you begin to find the common concepts beneath the different words, and that is what makes it possible to translate the concepts from one language to another. Analogously, beneath different social laws we find common human moral laws. Jewish, Indian, Chinese, Greek, Roman, Arabic, Babylonian, and Persian cultures have quite different mores; but Moses, Buddha, Confucius, Socrates, Cicero, Muhammad, Hammurabi, and Zoroaster have very similar morals. (See the Appendix to C.S. Lewis's The *Abolition of Man* for a short but instructive survey of some of these deep cross-cultural similarities in morality.)

(3) The Argument from Social Conditioning

The third argument for relativism is similar to the second but is more psychological than anthropological. It is also supposedly based on a scientifically verifiable fact: the fact that your society conditions values in you. For example, if you have been brought up in a Hindu society, you will have Hindu values. The origin of values thus seems to be human minds themselves—parents and teachers—rather than something objective to human minds. And what comes from human subjects is subjective, like the rules of baseball, even though they may be made public, universally known, and agreed to.

Reply

(a) This argument, like the previous one, also confuses values with value opinions. Perhaps society conditions value-opinions in us, but that does not mean that society conditions values in us— unless values are nothing but value opinions. But that is precisely the point at issue, the conclusion; it cannot also be the premise without begging the question.

(b) There is also a false assumption in this argument: that whatever we learn from society is subjective and man-made. That is not true. We learn the rules of baseball from our society, but we also learn the rules of multiplication from our society. The rules of baseball are subjective and man made, but the rules of multiplication are not. (The language systems and number systems in which we express the rules are man-made, of course.) The mind creates rather than discovers the rules of baseball, but the mind discovers rather than creates the rules of multiplication. So, the fact that we learn any given law or value from our society does not prove that it is subjective.

(c) Finally, the expressed premise of the argument is also false. Not all value opinions are the result of our social conditioning. For if they were, then there could never be any nonconformity to society based on moral values. There could only be rebellions of force, not of principle. But, in fact there are many principled nonconformists. They did not derive their values wholly from their society, since they disagree with their society about values. The existence of nonconformists shows the presence of some trans-social origin of values.

(4) The Argument from Freedom

A fourth argument is that moral relativism guarantees freedom while absolutism threatens it. How can you be wholly free if you are not free to create your own values? In fact our Supreme Court has declared that we have a fundamental right to define the mystery of life and the meaning of existence! (This is either the most fundamental of all rights, if it is right, or the most fundamental of all follies, if it is wrong. This is either the wisest or the stupidest thing the Court has ever written.) I think divine providence must have a dark sense of humor. This was the *Casey* decision. Do you remember what Casey did in the poem "Casey at the Bat"?

Reply

(a) The most effective reply to the argument from freedom is often an ad hominem. Say to the person who demands the right to freely create his own values that you too demand that right, and that the value system you have chosen to create is one in which his opinions have no weight at all, or one in which you are God and rightly demand his total obedience. He will quickly protest, in the name of truth and justice, thus showing that he really does believe in these two objective values after all. If he does not do this, and protests merely in the name of his alternative value system, which he has "freely" created, then his protest against your selfishness and megalomania is no better than your protest against his justice and truth. And then the "argument" comes down to not who is right, but who is stronger. When right disappears, might replaces it. And that is hardly a situation that guarantees freedom!

(b) A second refutation of the argument from freedom is that freedom cannot create values because it presupposes them. Arguing for subjective freedom must presuppose objective values. First, because the relativist's argument that relativism guarantees freedom assumes that freedom is really valuable. (Thus, there is at least one objective value: subjective freedom.) Second, if freedom is really good, it must be freedom from something really bad. Third, the advocate of freedom will almost always insist that freedom be granted to all, not just some, thus presupposing the real value of justice, or equality, or the Golden Rule.

(c) But, the simplest refutation of the argument is experiential. Experience shows us that we are free to create alternative mores, like socially acceptable rules for speech, clothing, eating, or driving. We are not, however, free to create another alternative set of morals, like justifying rape, murder, or treason, or forbidding justice, charity, or loyalty. We can no more create a new moral value than we can create a new primary color, a new arithmetic, or a new universe. Never happened, never will.

And if we could create "new" values, they would no longer be moral values, just invented rules of our game. We would not feel bound in conscience to honor them, or guilty when we transgressed them. If we were free to create "Thou shalt murder" or "Thou shalt not murder" as we are free to create "Thou shalt play nine innings" or "Thou shalt play six innings," we would no more feel guilty about murder than about playing six innings. As a matter of fact, we all do feel bound by fundamental moral values. We experience our freedom of will to choose to obey them or disobey them, but we also experience our lack of freedom to change them into their opposites, to "creatively" make hatred good or charity evil. Try it; you just can't do it. All you can do is to refuse the whole moral order, you cannot make another. You can choose to rape, but you cannot experience a moral obligation to rape.

(5) The Argument from Tolerance

Perhaps the most common argument against moral absolutism today is the argument from tolerance: that moral absolutism is "intolerant" while moral relativism is "tolerant." Tolerance is one of the few non-controversial values today; nearly everyone accepts it. So it is a powerful selling point for any theory or practice that can claim it. What of relativism's claim to tolerance?

I see no less than 8 fallacies in this popular argument.

(a) First, tolerance is a quality of people, not of ideas. Ideas can be confused, fuzzy, ill defined, or flexible, but this does not make them tolerant any more than clarity or exactness makes them intolerant. If a carpenter tolerates ³⁄₁₆ inch deviation from plumb, he is three times more tolerant than one who tolerates only ¹⁄₁₆ inch, but he is no less clear. One teacher (e.g. Marx) may tolerate no dissent from his fuzzy, ill-defined views, while another (e.g. Socrates) may tolerate much dissent from his clearly defined views.

(b) Second, suppose the relativist accepts the above distinction but still claims that absolutism (belief in universal, objective, unchanging moral laws) fosters personal intolerance of alternative views. However, a belief in universal, objective, and unchanging physical laws has not fostered personal intolerance of alternative views in the history of science. The sciences have progressed because of a tolerance of diverse and "heretical" views; yet, scientists have not concluded from this that they need to deny absolute physical laws. So, absolutism does not necessarily foster intolerance.

(c) The relativist may argue that absolutism does foster intolerance because absolutes are hard and unyielding, and therefore the defender of them will tend to be like them. But, this is also a non sequitur. One may teach hard facts in a soft way or soft opinions in a hard way.

In fact, if the teacher is confident of his "hard" facts, and if he loves and believes in objective truth, there is much less temptation for him to be intolerant. If he believes that the truth itself will set you free, he does not arrogate to himself that godlike task.

(d) The simplest refutation of the argument from tolerance is its assumption that tolerance is good—really, objectively, universally, and absolutely good. If the relativist replies that he is not presupposing the objective value of tolerance, then he is demanding the imposition of his own subjective personal preference for tolerance; and that is surely more intolerant than the appeal to a universal, impersonal, objective moral law that commands tolerance.

(e) Not only does absolutism foster tolerance, relativism fosters intolerance. Why not be intolerant? Because tolerance feels better? But sometimes it doesn't. Because it is the popular consensus? But it often isn't. The relativist can appeal to no moral law as a dam against intolerance. We need such a dam because societies, like individuals, are notoriously fickle. What else will deter a humane and humanistic Germany from turning to an inhumane Nazi morality of racism, or a now- tolerant America from turning to a future intolerance against any group it decides to disenfranchise? It is unborn babies today; it will be born babies tomorrow. It was homosexuals yesterday, it is homophobes today, and it may be homosexuals again tomorrow. The same moral absolutism that most homosexuals fear because it is not tolerant of their behavior is their only secure protection against intolerance of their persons.

(f) If we examine the essential meaning of the concept of tolerance, we will find that it presupposes a moral objectivism. For we do not tolerate goods, we tolerate evils in order to prevent worse evils. A doctor tolerates nausea brought on by chemotherapy in his cancer patient to prevent death; a society tolerates smoking and private drunkenness to preserve privacy and freedom. Tolerance "discriminates" between good and evil as much as intolerance does; more than intolerance does.

(g) The advocate of tolerance faces a dilemma when it comes to cross-cultural tolerance. Most cultures throughout history have put a very high price on tolerance. Some have even considered it a moral weakness. Should we tolerate this intolerance? If so, then the tolerant subjectivist had better stop bad-mouthing the Spanish Inquisition. But, if we should not tolerate intolerance, then why not? Because tolerance is really good and the Inquisition was really evil? In that case we are back in moral absolutism. We are presupposing and using a universal, objective, trans-cultural value. Well, then, what if the relativist says we should be tolerant only because our consensus is for tolerance? But, history's consensus is against it. Why impose ours? Is that not culturally intolerant?

(h) Finally, there is a logical non sequitur in the relativist's argument. Even if the belief in absolute moral values did cause intolerance, it does not follow that such values do not exist. The belief that the cop on the beat is sleeping may cause a mugger to be intolerant to his victims, but it does not follow that the cop is not asleep.

(6) The Argument from Situations and Motives

A sixth argument for relativism is that situations are so diverse, complex, and unpredictable that it is unreasonable and unrealistic to hold universal moral norms. Even killing can be good, if war is necessary for peace. Theft can be good, if you steal a weapon from a madman. Lying can be good, if you are a Dutchman hiding Jews from the Nazis.

The argument is essentially this: morality is determined by situations, and situations are relative, therefore morality is relative.

A closely related argument can be considered together with this one: that morality is relative because it is determined by subjective motives. We all blame a man for attempted murder, even though the deed was not done, simply because his motive is bad. We do not morally blame a man for accidental killing if there was nothing bad in his motive (e.g. if he gave sugar candy to a child he had no way of knowing was seriously diabetic).

The argument is essentially that morality is determined by motive, and motive is subjective, therefore morality is subjective.

Both the situationist and the motivationist conclude against moral absolutes: the situationist because he finds morality relative to the situation, the motivationist because he finds morality relative to the motive.

Reply

(a) The argument confuses *conditioning* and *determining*. Morality is indeed conditioned, or partly determined, by both situations and motives; but, it is not wholly determined by them. Traditional, common sense morality claims that there are three "moral determinants," three factors that influence whether a specific act is morally good or bad: the nature of the act itself, the motive, and the situation; or what you do, why you do it, and when, where, and how you do it.

It is true that doing the right thing for the wrong motive or in the wrong situation is not good. Giving money to the poor is a good deed, but doing it to show off is the wrong motive. Making love to your wife is good, but not when it is medically dangerous.

A good life is like a good work of art. A good work of art requires *all* its essential elements to be good. A good story must have a good plot, good characterization, a good theme, and a good style. It can be ruined by serious defect in any one of its essential dimensions. A good life requires that you do the right thing (the deed itself) and for the right reason (motive) and in the right way (the situation). No one of these can substitute for the other.

(b) And there must first *be* a deed before it can be qualified by subjective motives or relative situations. And that is surely a morally relevant factor too.

(c) And situations, though relative, are objective, not subjective. And motives, though subjective, come under universal moral absolutes: they can be recognized as intrinsically and universally good or evil. The will to help the good is always good; the will to harm them is always evil. So even situationism is an objective morality and even motivationism (or subjectivism) is a universal morality.

(d) In fact, we find that the vast majority of people today who say they no longer believe in any universal objective moral absolutes still believe in the universal subjective obligation to have good motives, such as moral honesty. Have you ever met anyone who believed it was good for anyone to deliberately disobey their own conscience?

(e) Furthermore, subjective motives are naturally connected with objective deeds. There are some deeds, like rape, that are incompatible with good motives, and other motives, like goodwill, that naturally produce good deeds (the *works* of charity).

(f) And the fact that the same principles must be applied differently to different situations (e.g. just war theory changes in a nuclear age) does not undermine these principles but presupposes them. Flexible applications of a standard presuppose a rigid standard. If the standard were as flexible as the situation, it would not be a standard. If the ruler with which you measure the length of a twisting alligator were as twisting as the alligator, you could not measure with it.

The distinction between deed and motive also helps answer the concern about tolerance. Moral absolutists need not be intolerant and "judgmental" about motives, which we do not know; only about deeds, which we do know. When Jesus said, "Judge not,' he surely meant "Do not claim to judge hearts and motives, which only God can know," rather than "Do not judge deeds, do not morally discriminate bullying from defending, robbery from charity." In fact, only the moral absolutist, and not the relativist, can condemn "judgmentalism" (of motive) and intolerance (of persons). The relativist can condemn only absolutism.

THE ARGUMENTS FOR ABSOLUTISM

Merely refuting all the arguments for relativism does not refute relativism itself. We need some positive arguments for absolutism as well. Here are five.

(1) The Pragmatic Argument from Consequences

If the relativist argues against absolutism from its supposed consequences of intolerance, we can argue against relativism from its real consequences. Consequences are at least clues, relevant signs. Good morality should have good consequences and bad morality bad ones.

It is very obvious that the main consequence of moral relativism is the removal of moral deterrence. Thus either all deterrence to immoral behavior is gone, and society collapses into chaos, or else the outer deterrent replaces the inner one: when conscience dies, cops multiply. The social consequence of moral relativism is either chaos or a police state.

Just as the consequences of "Do The Right Thing" are doing the right thing, so the consequences of "If It Feels Good, Do it" are doing whatever feels good. It takes no Ph.D. to see that. In fact, it takes a Ph.D. to miss it. *All* immoral deeds and attitudes feel good; that's why we do them. If sin didn't seem like fun, we'd all be saints.

Relativism never produced a saint. That is the practical argument against relativism.

The same goes for societies. Relativism never produced a good society, only bad ones— "bad" not just by moral standards but by pragmatic standards. Compare the happiness, stability, and longevity of societies founded on the principles of moral relativists like Mussolini and Mao Zedong with societies founded on the principles of moral absolutists like Moses and Confucius. Confucius' society lasted 2100 years. Hitler's "Thousand-year Reich" lasted twelve.

If you classify Mussolini and Hitler as absolutists, you do not know much about Fascism. I wonder whether Justice Kennedy would have written the "mystery" passage in the Casey decision (quoted above) if he knew the following quotation from Mussolini:

> "Everything I have said and done in these last years is relativism. . . . If relativism signifies contempt for fixed categories and men who claim to be the bearers of an objective, immortal truth . . . then there is nothing more relativistic than Fascistic attitudes and activity. . . . From the fact that all ideologies are of equal value, that all ideologies are mere fictions, the modern relativist infers that everybody has the right to create for himself his own ideology and to attempt to enforce it with all the energy of which he is capable." (Benito Mussolini, *Diuturna* pp. 374–77, quoted in Helmut Kuhn, *Freedom Forgotten and Remembered* Chapel Hill, North Carolina: University of North Carolina Press, 1943, pp. 17–18.)

(2) The Argument from Tradition

Many relativists argue against absolutism because they think it is connected with snobbery. It is exactly the opposite. Absolutism is *traditional* morality, and tradition is egalitarianism extended into history. Chesterton called tradition "the democracy of the dead": extending the franchise to that most powerless of classes, those disenfranchised not by accident of birth but by accident of death. Tradition counters the small and arrogant oligarchy of the living, those who just happen to be walking around this planet today.

To be a relativist, you must be a snob, at least on this centrally important issue. For you stand in a tiny minority, almost wholly concentrated in one culture, the modern West (i.e. European, democratic, industrialized, urbanized, university-educated, secularized, post-Christian society). To be a relativist, you must believe that nearly all human beings in history have ordered their lives by an illusion.

Even in societies like ours that are dominated by relativistic "experts," popular opinion tends to moral absolutism. Like Communists, relativists often pretend to be the party of "the people" while in fact scorning the people's philosophy. In fact, for a generation now a minority of relativistic, media-empowered elitists have been branding the traditional morality of popular opinion as elitism!

But any argument from consensus can only be probable. As the medieval philosophers well knew, "the argument from (human) authority is the weakest of all arguments." The fact that most people today are surprised by that statement is an indication of the success of the modern elitist's indoctrination. They have been taught that the Middle Ages, being religious, were authoritarian while modern civilization is rational. But, the truth is almost exactly the opposite. Medieval thinkers were rational to a fault, while modern philosophy since the "Enlightenment" has attacked reason in a dozen different ways and preferred the authority of passion, pragmatism, politics, or power.

(3)The Argument from Moral Experience

This argument is probably the simplest and strongest argument for moral absolutism. In fact, it seems strained to call it an argument; it is more like primary data. It is that the first and foundational moral experience is always absolutistic. Only later in the life of the individual or the society does sophistication sometimes suggest moral relativism. Each of us remembers from early childhood experience what it feels like to be morally obligated, to be in the presence of real right and wrong, to bump up against an unyielding moral truth like a wall.

We still know that moral absolutism is true by experience. Our attempts to explain moral conscience as a feeling are refuted not by philosophical argument but immediate experience. For instance, say that last night you promised your friend you would help him early the next morning to move his furniture from his apartment, which he has to evacuate by noon. But, you were up till 3 AM. and when your alarm rings at seven you are very tired. You experience two things: the desire to sleep and the obligation to get up. The two are generically different: you experience no obligation to sleep and no desire to get up. You are moved in one way by your own desire to sleep, and in a totally different way by what you think you ought to do. Your feelings and desires appear from the inside out, so to speak, but your moral conscience appears from the outside in. The desire to sleep is within you, and this may move you to the external deed of shutting off the alarm and creeping back to bed. Instead, if you get up to fulfill your promise, it will be because you chose to respond to a wholly different kind of thing: the perceived moral quality of the deed of fulfilling your promise, as opposed to the perceived moral quality of refusing it. What you perceive as right or obligatory (getting up) *pulls* you from without, from itself, from its own nature. The desires you feel as attractive (going back to sleep) *pushes* you from within, from your own nature. The moral obligation moves you as an end, as a final cause, from above and ahead, so to speak; the desire moves you as a source, as an efficient cause, from below and behind, so to speak.

All this is primary data, the most fundamental moral experience. It can be denied, but only as some strange philosophy might deny the reality immediately perceived by our senses. Moral relativism is to moral experience what the teaching of Buddhism is to matter or Mary Baker Eddy's "Christian Science" is to pain, sickness, and death: it tells us they are illusions to be overcome by faith. Moral absolutism is hard-headed, data-driven, and empirical; moral relativism is a dreamy, mystical dogma of faith.

(4) The Ad Hominem Argument

Even the relativist reacts with a moral protest when treated immorally. The man who appeals to the relativistic principle of "I gotta be me" to justify breaking his promise of fidelity to his own wife will then break his fidelity to his relativistic principle when his new wife uses that principle to justify leaving him for another man. This is not exceptional but typical. It looks like the origin of relativism is more personal than philosophical, more like hypocrisy than hypothesis.

The contradiction between theory and practice is evident even in the relativist's act of teaching relativism. Why do relativists teach and write? To convince the world that relativism is right and absolutism is wrong? *Really* right and *really* wrong? Then there is a real right and wrong. If not, then there is nothing wrong with being an absolutist and nothing right about being a relativist.

So why do relativists write and teach? Really, from all the effort they have put into preaching their gospel of liberating humanity from the false and foolish repressions of moral absolutism, one would have thought that they believed their sermons. Apparently, there is a hypocrisy hiding here again.

(5) The Argument from Moral Language

A very obvious argument is the one used by C.S. Lewis at the very beginning of *Mere Christianity*. It is based on the observation that people quarrel. They do not merely fight, but argue about right and wrong. People act as if they believed in objectively real and universally binding moral principles. If nothing but subjective desires and passions were involved, it would merely be a contest of strength between competing persons or between competing passions within a person. (If I am more hungry than tired, I will eat, if I am more tired than hungry, I will sleep.) But we say things like "That's not fair", or "What right do you have to that?" If relativism were true, moral argument would be as stupid as arguing about feelings: "I feel great.", "No! I feel terrible!"

In fact, the daily moral language that praises, blames, counsels, and commands, would be strictly meaningless if relativism were true. We do not praise or blame non-moral agents like machines. When the Coke machine "steals" our money without giving us a Coke, we do not argue with it, call it a sinner, or tell it to go to Confession. We kick it. So when many of our psychologists tell us that we are only very complex machines, they are telling us that morality is only very complex kicking.

This is so absurd it hardly deserves an argument. It deserves something more like a spanking. (Which would only be to practice what they preach.)

Moral language is meaningful, not meaningless. We all know how to use it, and we do. Relativism cannot explain that simple fact.

THE CAUSE AND CURE OF RELATIVISM

This is the most important point of all. The real source of moral relativism is not any argument, and therefore, its cure is also not any argument. Neither philosophy nor science nor logic nor common sense nor experience has refuted traditional moral absolutism. Not reason but the abdication of reason is the source of moral relativism. Relativism is not rational, it is rationalization. It is not the conclusion of a rational argument, it is the rationalization of a prior passion, the repudiation of the principle that passions should be evaluated by reason and controlled by will. That is the virtue Plato and Aristotle called self-control. It is not just one of the four cardinal virtues, but a necessary ingredient in every virtue. This classical assumption is almost the definition of civilization. But romanticists, Freudians, existentialists, deconstructionists, and others have convinced many people today that it is unhealthy, repressive, and 'inauthentic." If we embrace the opposite principle and let passion govern reason or rationalization substitute for honesty, there is little hope for civilization, much less for morality.

Sexual passion is obviously the strongest and most attractive of the passions. It is, therefore, also the most addictive and the most blinding. So there could hardly be a more powerful way to undermine our moral knowledge and our moral life than the Sexual Revolution. Already, our demand for sexual "freedom" has overridden one of nature's strongest instincts, motherhood. A million mothers a year in America alone pay hired killers, called healers or physicians, to kill their own unborn daughters and sons. How could this happen? None of our ancestors would have believed it. It happened only because abortion is driven by sexual motives. Abortion is backup birth control, and birth control is the demand to have sex without having babies.

Divorce is a second example of the power of the Sexual Revolution to undermine basic moral principles. Suppose there were some other practice, not connected with sex, which had the same three effects as divorce: first, betraying the person you had solemnly sworn to love for the rest of your life; second, abusing the vulnerable children you had procreated and promised to protect, deeply scarring their souls and making it far more difficult for them ever to attain happy lives or marriages; and third, harming, undermining, and destroying your society's future (for divorce is the suicide of the family, and the family is society's basic building block). Would not such a practice be universally condemned? Yet, that is what divorce is, and it is nearly universally accepted. Betrayal of persons and promises is universally condemned—unless it is for sex. Not causing misery, not doing harm, especially to children, especially to your own children—this is universally condemned, unless it interferes with your sexual freedom. Contributing to your society's destruction is never condoned, unless it would interfere with your sexual happiness. The rest of traditional morality is still widely believed and taught, even in soap operas and movies. No one justifies nuclear war, terrorism, insider trading, torture, the Mafia, or even pollution. The driving force of moral relativism today seems almost always exclusively sexual.

Why this is so and what we can do about it are two questions that demand much more time and thought than we have available here. But, if you want a very short guess at an answer to both, here is the best I can do.

A secularist has only one substitute left for God, only one experience in a desacralized world that still gives him something like the mystical thrill of self-transcendence, the ecstasy (literally, "standing-outside-self") that God designed all souls for, and which we cannot help longing for until we have it. Unless he is a surfer, that experience is going to be sex.

We are designed for far more than happiness. We are designed for joy. Aquinas writes, with simple logic, "Man cannot live without joy. That is why one deprived of spiritual joys must go over to carnal pleasures."

Drugs and alcohol attract because they claim to feed the same need. They lack the ontological greatness of sex, but they provide the same kind of semi-mystical thrill: the transcendence of self-consciousness, reason, and responsibility. I do not mean this merely as moral condemnation, but as psychological understanding. In fact, though it may sound shocking, I think the addict is closer to the ultimate truth than the mere moralist. He is looking for the very best thing in some of the very worst places. His demand for a state in which he transcends morality is very wrong, but it is also very right. For we are designed for something beyond morality, something in which morality will be transformed: mystical union with God, a mystical marriage. That is not a pale image of sex; sex is a pale image of that. Moral absolutists must never forget that morality, though absolute, is not ultimate, not our *summum bonum*, our greatest good. Mount Sinai is not the promised land; Mount Zion is. And in the New Jerusalem, what finally happens as the last chapter in human history, according to the only book that tells the whole story, is a wedding, between the Lamb and His Bride. Deprived of that Jerusalem, we must buy into Babylon. If we do not worship God, we will worship idols, for we are by nature worshippers.

Finally, what is the cure? It must be stronger medicine than philosophy. I can give you only three words to answer the last, most practical question of all. And they are totally unoriginal. For they are not my philosophical arguments, but God's Biblical demands: repent, fast, and pray. Confess, sacrifice, and adore. Nothing else can save our civilization except saints.

Please be one.

III

LAW AND PUBLIC MORALITY

5

Science, Law, and the "Culture of Death"

Charles E. Rice

The moral question of the proper relationship between science and law is not new. Historically, science and law seem to compete for opposing goods. Science strives for ingenuity and progress while law for restrictions and tradition. The effort to make science more legal, however, misses the point. A moral science begins with ethical scientists who are willing to place the dignity of the human being above the goals of research and progress. Pope John Paul II speaks of a "culture of death" that has made human life a good instrumental unto science and progress. What modern culture needs to remedy this fallacy is Christ-centered scientists, whose work serves the absolute good of human life and the glory of God. Good people more than good laws will make modern science moral.

SHOULD LAW LIMIT SCIENCE?

This question involves new manifestations of a long-standing tendency of some scientists to liberate themselves from ethical norms. In notable cases, the law has condoned, if not mandated, that liberation:

"New treatments for malaria and vaccines for typhus . . . were developed in [Nazi] concentration camp experiments. And . . . rescue services will today determine how long a person can survive in cold water using data figured out at Dachau and Buchenwald concentration camps, where scientists systematically immersed victims in freezing water until they died. In Tuskegee, Alabama . . . 399 syphilitic African Americans were deliberately not treated for their condition over the course of 40 years (from 1932 to 1972), simply so that medical scientists could

study the progression of the untreated disease. . . . In the 1950s . . . children at a
school for the mentally retarded in Waltham, Massachusetts, were fed radioactive
oatmeal in an experiment . . . to trace the path of radioactive food through the
digestive tract. Neither they, nor their parents, gave consent."[1]

Embryonic stem cell research and cloning are perhaps the most controversial issues that currently pose the question of whether science should be
limited by law. On August 9, 2001, President Bush announced a compromise
policy under which researchers using federal money may work with embryonic stem cell lines established before that date but may not generate new
lines after that date.[2] That prohibition does not prevent the use of federal
money for research on stem cells obtained from aborted fetuses rather than
from embryos.[3] In March, 2002, the National Institutes of Health ruled that
federally financed researchers could study new stem cell lines—and even
derive them from embryos—provided that they do not commingle their federal and private money.[4] Recent research indicates that embryonic stem cells
have limited, if any, potential for the treatment of cancer, diabetes,
Alzheimer's, and Parkinson's; and that superior results are likely from the use
of adult stem cells derived from bone marrow and stem cells derived from
umbilical cord blood.[5] Those alternative sources do not raise the ethical
problems presented by the derivation of stem cells from embryos.[6]

On the cloning issue, H.R. 234, sponsored by Congressmen Dave Weldon,
M.D. (R-FL) and Bart Stupak (D-MI) would ban all human cloning.[7] Unlike
Weldon-Stupak, S. 303, introduced by Senators Hatch and Feinstein (S. 303)
would ban only "reproductive cloning" in which the clone is intended to be
implanted in a woman's uterus and carried to birth. S. 303 would allow "therapeutic cloning," in which the clone is intended for research purposes. "In
reproductive cloning, the early-stage embryo that results is nurtured to the
point that it can be implanted in the womb of a surrogate mother to produce
an infant. In therapeutic cloning, the development of the resulting primitive
embryo or 'blastocyst' is halted as soon as a cluster of stem cells develops.
The stem cells then are harvested for research purposes."[8] In "therapeutic
cloning," of course, all of the cloned embryos are deliberately killed. The
Hatch/Feinstein bill allows somatic cell nuclear transfer, which is cloning.
The bill would ban the *birth* of cloned babies while allowing use of cloning
to create human embryos for life-saving research. The bill makes it a crime
to let an unfrozen cloned human embryo live past 14 days,[9] a provision that
would put the federal government in the position of mandating the death of
innocent human beings before birth.

So when should science be limited by law? In rejecting "the principle of
the unlimited freedom of scientific research," Pope John Paul II said, "On the
one hand . . . it is necessary to admit the right of sciences to apply their own
methods of research, but, on the other, one cannot agree with the declara-

tion that the province of research is subject to no restrictions. The fundamental distinction between good and evil sets up one boundary. This distinction is known by the human conscience. One can say that the autonomy of science ends where the honest conscience of the scientist admits evil—evil in method, product, or effect."[10]

As Thomas Aquinas taught, the human law should not try to "forbid all vices, from which the virtuous abstain, but only the more grievous vices, from which it is possible for the majority to abstain, and chiefly those that are to the hurt of others, without the prohibition of which human society could not be maintained: thus human law prohibits murder, theft, and suchlike."[11] The law should "lead men to virtue, not suddenly but gradually," lest the law be "despised" and "greater evils" result.[12] Aquinas, here as elsewhere, writes from a realistic view of human nature. "Human law," he says, "does not lay upon the multitude of imperfect men the burdens of those who are already virtuous, viz., that they should abstain from all evil. Otherwise, these imperfect ones, being unable to bear such precepts, would break out into yet greater evils: thus it is written . . . (*Matthew*. ix. 17) that if new wine (i.e. precepts of a perfect life) is put into old bottles (i.e. into imperfect men) the bottles break, and the wine runneth out (i.e. the precepts are despised) and those men, from contempt, break out into evils worse still."[13] The human law therefore "'allows and leaves unpunished many things that are punished by Divine Providence.'"[14]

The 1987 *Instruction on Bioethics* is still pertinent to the discussion of the proper use of law as a limitation on science. The Church claims no "particular competence in the area of the experimental sciences."[15] However, she does claim that "science and technology require, for their own intrinsic meaning, an unconditional respect for the fundamental criteria of the moral law: that is to say, they must be at the service of the human person, of his inalienable rights and his true and integral good according to the design and will of God. . . . [S]cience without conscience can only lead to man's ruin."[16] The document continues:

> [T]he human body cannot be considered as a mere complex of tissues, organs and functions, nor can it be evaluated in the same way as the body of animals; rather it is a constitutive part of the person who manifests and expresses himself through it. The natural moral law expresses and lays down the purposes, rights, and duties which are based upon the bodily and spiritual nature of the human person. Therefore, this law cannot be thought of as simply a set of norms on the biological level; rather it must be defined as the rational order whereby man is called by the Creator to direct and regulate his life and actions and in particular to make use of his own body. . . . [A]rtificial interventions on procreation and on the origin of human life . . . are not to be rejected on the ground that they are artificial. But, they must be given a moral evaluation in reference to the dignity of the human person.[17]

These concepts are echoed in the Catechism of the Catholic Church:

> It is an illusion to claim moral neutrality in scientific research and its applications. On the other hand, guiding principles cannot be inferred from simple technical efficiency, or from the usefulness accruing to some at the expense of others or, even worse, from prevailing ideologies. Science and technology by their very nature require unconditional respect for fundamental moral criteria. They must be at the service of the human person, of his inalienable rights, of his true and integral good, in conformity with the plan and the will of God.[18]

In its chapter III, on Moral and Civil Law, the 1987 *Instruction on Bioethics* acknowledged that the law "must sometimes tolerate, for the sake of public order, things which it cannot forbid without a greater evil resulting. However, the inalienable rights of the person must be recognized and respected by civil society and the political authority." The *Instruction* specified two general rights the law must protect:

a) every human being's right to life and physical integrity from the moment of conception until death;
b) the rights of the family and of marriage as an institution and, in this area, the child's right to be conceived, brought into the world and brought up by his parents.

With respect to the "right to life and physical integrity," the *Instruction* said, "The law must provide appropriate penal sanctions for every deliberate violation of the child's rights. The law cannot tolerate—indeed it must expressly forbid—that human beings, even at the embryonic stage, should be treated as objects of experimentation, be mutilated or destroyed with the excuse that they are superfluous or incapable of developing normally."

On "the rights of the family and of marriage," the *Instruction* said, "Civil law cannot grant approval to techniques of artificial procreation. . . . cannot legalize the donation of gametes between persons who are not legitimately united in marriage . . . . [and] must also prohibit, by virtue of the support which is due to the family, embryo banks, *post mortem* insemination, and 'surrogate motherhood.'"

The *Instruction* also mandated that, with respect to "morally unacceptable civil laws," "'conscientious objection' . . . must be supported and recognized."

THE ENLIGHTENMENT AND THE ROOTS OF THE CULTURAL WAR

The *Instruction on Bioethics* thus enumerates a few important ways in which the law should limit science. The principles of the *Instruction* are applicable to present issues such as embryonic stem cell research and cloning. We should recognize, however, that there is no practical chance of enacting today, on either the federal or state level, the sort of specific legal restrictions prescribed by the *Instruction*. This is so because we are living through what Francis Canavan, S.J., called, "the fag end of the Enlightenment."[19] American culture today is what John Paul II aptly called "a culture of death"[20] based on Enlightenment premises.

The self proclaimed Enlightenment of the past three centuries has been the effort of numerous philosophers and politicians to build a society without God. The premises of the Enlightenment are secularism, relativism, and individualism. In its secularism, the Enlightenment tells us that reason cannot know anything about God or about objective moral truth. It provides, for example, the rationale for the philosophy of "speciesism," which is prejudice against persons who are not members of the species, *Homo sapiens*, and to conclude that "killing . . . a chimpanzee is worse than the killing of a gravely defective human who is not a person."[21]

In its relativism, the Enlightenment has some form of legal positivism as its jurisprudence. If, as Hans Kelsen said, "Justice is an irrational ideal"[22], then no law can be rationally criticized as unjust, still less declared void on that ground. Thus, Kelsen acknowledged that the laws of the Nazi regime were valid law, regardless of their content, because they were enacted by the prescribed procedures and were effective.[23] American jurisprudence owes much of its present character to the similarly positivistic "legal realism" of Oliver Wendell Holmes,[24] who defined truth as "the majority vote of the nation that could lick all others,"[25] and who said, "I see no reason for attributing to man a significance different in kind from that which belongs to a baboon or a grain of sand."[26]

In its individualism, the Enlightenment postulates that human persons began in a mythical "state of nature" in which they were not social but "sociable."[27] They had no inherent relation to others, but rather freely chose to live in a society and submit to its laws. This is the origin of the "pro-choice" movement today. A mother has no relation to the child she is carrying unless she consents. As theories of the social contract were described by Cardinal Ratzinger, "when the common reference to values and ultimately to God is lost, society will then appear merely as an ensemble of individuals placed side by side, and the contract which ties them together will necessarily be perceived as an accord among those who have the power to impose their will on others."[28] The autonomous individual of the Enlightenment detaches conscience from any relation to objective truth. Freedom is "understood as the absolute right to self-determination on the basis of one's own convictions."[29]

In Enlightenment thinking, the state no longer derives its authority from God and therefore is no longer limited by natural or divine law. "The Declaration of the Rights of Man at the end of the eighteenth century," wrote

Hannah Arendt, "was a turning point in history. It meant nothing more nor less than that from then on Man, and not God's command or the customs of history, should be the source of Law."[30]

The fading but still dominant Enlightenment culture is not receptive to the legislative proposals envisioned by the *Instruction on Bioethics*. In addition, there is no practical chance of adopting a constitutional amendment to restore personhood to the unborn child so as to prevent his execution by abortion in any case.

The culture must be changed in a pro-life direction if the law is to extend coherent protection to a right to life. The advocacy of uncompromising, pro-life legislation can itself be a catalyst for cultural change. Legal and cultural change goes together. So we ought to support, for instance, the Weldon bill to ban all human cloning, which has a strong chance of passing. And we should support the proposals recommended by the *Instruction on Bioethics*. Such legislative efforts, however, may have their primary utility in fostering a cultural change of attitude, building a "culture of life" from the ground up.

A CENTRAL ISSUE: THE MORALITY OF SEX

The decisive—and commonly overlooked—cultural issue here is contraception. William Bennett, in the various editions of his Index of Cultural Indicators, has spelled out the cultural and moral meltdown which began in the 1960s.[31] What happened in the 1960s to trigger that meltdown? One event was the Supreme Court's decree, in the school prayer cases, that government must be neutral on the existence of God.[32] Generations of children have graduated from the public school system without ever seeing the state, in the person of the teacher, acknowledge a standard of right and wrong higher than itself. Basically, every child has been enrolled in Legal Positivism 101.

The second event of the 1960s was the marketing of the contraceptive pill. As Pope Paul VI taught in *Humanae Vitae*, "contraception separates the unitive and procreative aspects of sex."[33] John Paul II emphasized also that the contracepting couple claim "a power which belongs solely to God: the power to decide, in *a final analysis*, the coming into existence of a human person."[34] Contracting couples also "manipulate" and degrade human sexuality and with it themselves and their married partner by altering its value of 'total' self-giving."[35]

"Nature is manipulated every day as rivers are dammed to store water; plants and animals are bred to supply food, fibres, companionship, and sport; and the natural progress of disease is checked by surgery and drugs. So people ask: *"What is the difference between removing a diseased appendix and tying fallopian tubes, or between taking an antibiotic and taking the contraceptive pill?"* One difference is easily explained. Appendices are only removed when they become diseased. Antibiotics are taken to kill dangerous micro-organisms. Such therapeutic procedures restore patients to health—by destroying pathological bacteria or removing malfunctioning bodily parts. Contraceptives function in a totally different way. Instead of removing a malfunction they actually produce one. Contraceptives turn normal fertility into an abnormal, sterile state. They impair the functions of healthy reproductive organs. Contraceptives damage the bodies of those who use them and they are taken for that express purpose. Contraceptives have more in common with poisons or pesticides than with operations and medications directed against disease."[36]

Contraception is the great unmentionable in the pro-life movement and in Catholic churches. Mainstream "pro-life" organizations and leaders, including notably the National Right to Life Committee, refuse to acknowledge contraception as a pro-life issue except to the extent that so-called contraceptives operate as abortifacients. Thus, Dr. & Mrs. John C. Willke state, "'Contraception is not a Right to Life issue, but I.U.D.'s, Norplant and 'Emergency Contraception' are referred to as contraceptives when, in fact, they are 'abortifacients.' Use the correct word."[37] Some pro-life organizations, including the American Life League, Catholics United for Life, Population Research Institute, and Human Life International accurately identify the acceptance of contraception as the decisive vice of the "culture of death." It will be impossible to build a culture of life and to define a sound relation between science and the law without rejecting contraception.

The cultural acceptance of contraception is the unacknowledged, but determinative factor in the rise of several otherwise mystifying phenomena of the "culture of death." A contraceptive society needs abortion as a back-up, a fail-safe contraceptive. Contraception accepts the premise that there is such a thing as a human life not worth living. That premise underlies abortion and euthanasia. Also, the practice of contraception has resulted in a "graying" of the population of the United States. The reduced number of workers, apart from immigrants, available to support the growing number of elderly persons has fueled pressure for quiet forms of euthanasia through "terminal sedation" and other techniques.

If the premises of contraception are true, if it is entirely up to the persons involved whether sex will have any relation to procreation, what reason other than the pragmatic or the aesthetic can be advanced for denying Freddy and Harry or Ginger and Sue, a marriage license? If we are concerned about teen-age promiscuity and divorce, perhaps we ought to reflect that one reason why, in the nature of things, sex is reserved for marriage and marriage is permanent is that sex has something to do with babies. But, if there is no inherent relation between sex and babies and if it is entirely up to us to decide whether there should be—why should sex be reserved for marriage and why should marriage be permanent? In *Humanae Vitae*, Paul

VI warned that if contraception were accepted, woman would come to be regarded as an object of pleasure and not as a person. At the University of Notre Dame and other bastions of the American Church, they laughed at Paul VI for that one. Today, when internet pornography sites are a bigger money maker than the major networks, nobody is laughing anymore.

In vitro fertilization is the reverse of contraception. Contraception involves the effort to seize the recreational, while deliberately frustrating the procreational aspects of sex. (In fact the contracepting couple gets neither because they reduce the conjugal act to an exercise in mutual masturbation). But the separation of the unitive and procreative aspects of sex is characteristic of *in vitro* fertilization no less than it is of contraception. A contraceptive society has no principled ground to reject *in vitro* and other reductions of self-generation to a laboratory process. And if, through contraception, man (of both sexes) assumes the right to decide whether, when, and how life shall begin; what logical line can be drawn short of embryonic stem cell research, cloning, and whatever other refinements may be over the horizon?

The law is limited in this area. Few legal restrictions are practical with respect to contraception. Unlike abortion, which involves murder which the law can never rightly allow in any case, contraception should be approached in an incremental fashion. To begin, a sound pro-life initiative would be to propose a prohibition of the distribution of contraceptives to minors, or at least distribution without specific parental consent. Such a proposal would end the practice of school-based clinics providing contraceptives to impressionable children without parental consent.

The development of early abortifacients and the growing practice of "terminal sedation" as a form of palliative care, have confirmed the reality that abortion and euthanasia are moving beyond the reach of the law. The dominant abortion of the near future, and increasingly of the present, will be accomplished by chemical and other abortifacient substances and devices. Abortion will become a truly private matter, affected only in the doctor's office. It will soon become nearly impossible to prove that an abortion has actually occurred. And some abortifacient drugs have legitimate uses other than abortion. If they are licensed for any use, it will be practically impossible for the law to prevent their use for abortion. Moreover, the prevalent definition of pregnancy over the past few decades as beginning at implantation of the child in the womb rather than at fertilization, clears the way for early abortifacients to be regarded as contraceptives. Similarly, in upholding state prohibitions of assisted suicide, the Supreme Court gave explicit approval of palliative care, even if it causes death, pursuant to the principle of the double effect.[38] Except in an aggravated case, the blunt instrument of the law will be unable to determine whether a physician's administration of "pain medication" is lawful palliative care or a homicidal "terminal sedation."

Numerous legislative proposals, on the federal and state levels, could be proposed to throw sand in the gears of the abortion industry without compromise of principle, including, for example, provisions to facilitate malpractice recovery from abortionists.[39] On the homosexual issue, we must draw a line in the sand against the conferral on "de facto unions," whether homo- or heterosexual, of the incidents or name of marriage.

Handing on the Gospel message in today's world is particularly arduous, mainly because our contemporaries are immersed in cultural contexts that are often alien to an inner spiritual dimension. In situations in which a materialist outlook prevails, one cannot escape the fact that, more than in any other historical period, there is a breakdown in the process of handing on moral and religious values between generations. This leads to a kind of incongruity between the Church and the contemporary world.[40] Several generations of Catholic school students have wasted their religion classes making collages. But, there is reason to hope that the resulting gap will be closed. "God is preparing a great springtime for Christianity," says John Paul, "and we can already see its first signs."[41] The answer to the many challenges posed by the "culture of death" is in the moral and social teachings of the Catholic Church.

In response to the secularism of the Enlightenment, John Paul II teaches that the cultural separation of conscience from any obligation of fidelity to the truth is a result of a more basic dichotomy, the separation of morality from faith. He insists on identifying the Lawgiver of the natural law. In response to the relativism of the Enlightenment, John Paul affirms that there is an objective moral standard. That standard, however, is not an abstraction or a slogan. It is a Person—Jesus Christ. In response to the individualism of the Enlightenment, John Paul says that Christ, the moral standard who is Truth, shows us on the crucifix that a human person can truly fulfill himself through self-gift, through the gift of self to others for love of God and man.

The task of the committed Catholic is to come out of the bomb shelters on contraception and other issues relating to law and science. A sound relation between the law and science can be restored only through the Truth who is Christ.

NOTES

1. Financial Times (London) July14, 2001, Body and Mind section, p. 2. See also Final Report, Tuskegee Syphilis Study Legacy Committee—May 20, 1996.

2. N.Y. Times, Dec. 12, 2002, p. A29.

3. Chicago Tribune (on line ed.), July 7, 2002.

4. N.Y. Times, Aug. 7, 2002, p. A1.

5. Washington Times, Dec. 31, 2002, p. A3; Joseph Perkins, Bad Science Behind Stem Cell Research, Wash. Times, Dec. 26, 2002, p. A16.

6. "A stem cell has been found in adults that can turn into every single tissue in the body. It might turn out to be the most important cell ever discovered.

"Until now, only stem cells from early embryos were thought to have such properties. If the finding is confirmed, it will mean cells from your own body could one day be turned into all sorts of perfectly matched replacement tissues and even organs.

"If so, there would be no need to resort to therapeutic cloning—cloning people to get matching stem cells from the resulting embryos. Nor would you have to genetically engineer embryonic stem cells (ESCs) to create a 'one cell fits all' line that does not trigger immune rejection. The discovery of such versatile adult stem cells will also fan the debate about whether embryonic stem-cell research is justified." New Scientist, Jan. 23, 2002.

7. H.R. 234 (108th Cong., 1st Sess.) provides:

§ 301. Definitions

"In this chapter:

"(1) HUMAN CLONING.—The term 'human cloning' means human asexual reproduction, accomplished by introducing nuclear material from one or more human somatic cells into a fertilized or unfertilized oocyte whose nuclear material has been removed or inactivated so as to produce a living organism (at any stage of development) that is genetically virtually identical to an existing or previously existing human organism.

"(2) ASEXUAL REPRODUCTION.—the term 'asexual reproduction' means reproduction not initiated by the union of oocyte and sperm.

"(3) SOMATIC CELL.—The term 'somatic cell' means a diploid cell (having a complete set of chromosomes) obtained or derived from a living or deceased human body at any stage of development.

"§ 302. Prohibition on human cloning

"(a) IN GENERAL.—It shall be unlawful for any person or entity, public or private, in or affecting interstate commerce, knowingly—

"(1) to perform or attempt to perform human cloning;

"(2) to participate in an attempt to perform human cloning; or

"(3) to ship or receive for any purpose an embryo produced by human cloning.

"(b) IMPORTATION.—It shall be unlawful for any person or entity, public or private, knowingly to import for any purpose an embryo produced by human cloning

8. Amy Fagan, Cloning Issue Again before Senate, Wash. Times, Jan. 13, 2003.

9. "(d) FOURTEEN-DAY RULE.—An unfertilized blastocyst shall not be maintained after more than 14 days from its first cell division, not counting any time during which it is stored at temperatures less than zero degrees centigrade." S.303 (108th Cong., 1st Sess.), Sec. 499A(d).

10. S.T., I, II, Q. 96, art. 1.

11. Pope John Paul II, Address to Rectors and Professors of Polish Universities, Aug. 30, 2001; 47 *The Pope Speaks* (Mar/Apr 2002), 78, 80–81.

12. S.T., I, II, Q. 96, art. 2.

13. Ibid.

14. Ibid.

15. Congregation for the Doctrine of the Faith, *Instruction on Respect for Human Life in Its Origin and on the Dignity of Procreation* (1987), Intro., No. 1.

16. *Ibid.*, Intro., No. 2.

17. *Ibid.*, Intro. No. 3.

18. Catechism of the Catholic Church, no. 2294.

19. Francis Canavan, S.J. "Commentary," *Catholic Eye*, Dec. 10, 1987, p.2.

20. *Evangelium Vitae* (1995), no. 28.

21. Peter Singer, Practical Ethics (1979), 97.

22. Hans Kelsen, "The Pure Theory of Law, Part I," 50 Law Quart. Rev. 474, 482 (1934).

23. Hans Kelsen, *Das Natuarrecht in der politischen Theorie* (F.M. Schmoelz, ed., 1963), 148, quoted in translation in F.A. Hayek, *Law, Legislation and Liberty* (1976), vol. 2, 56.

24. See Francis E. Lucey, S.J., "Natural Law and American Legal Realism: Their Respective Contributions to a Theory of Law in a Democratic Society," 30 Georgetown L.J., 493 (1942).

25. Oliver Wendell Holmes, *The Natural Law Collected Legal Papers* (1920< 310.

26. 2 *Holmes-Pollock Letters* (1942), 252; see discussion in William Kenealy, S.J., "The Majesty of the Law," 5 *Loyola Law Rev.* 101, 107–08 (1950); Charles E. Rice, *Beyond Abortion: The Theory and Practice of the Secular State* (1979), chs. 2 and 6.

27. See Heinrich Rommen, *The Natural Law* (1948), 75–109.

28. Joseph Ratzinger, "The Problem of Threats to Human Life," 36 *The Pope Speaks*, 334–35 (1991).

29. *Ibid.*

30. Hannah Arendt, *The Origins of Totalitarianism* (1966), 290.

31. See William J. Bennett, *Index of Leading Cultural Indicators* (1993).

32. See *Abington School District v. Schempp*, 374 U.S. 203, 215 (1963).

33. *Humanae Vitae*, no. 12.

34. Pope John Paul II, *Discourse*, Sept. 17, 1983; 28 *The Pope Speaks* 356, 356–57 (1983).

35. Pope John Paul II, *Familiaris Consortio* (1981), no. 32.

36. Les Hemingway, Contraception and Common Sense (Dr. Les Hemingway, Warrnambool Victoria 3280, Australia, 1997(, p. 1).

37. John C. Willke, M.D., and Barbara Willke, *Abortion: Questions and Answers* (2003), 344.

38. Vacco v. Quill, 521 U.S. 793, 807–08, n. 11 (1997).

39. See the enumeration of proposals in Charles E. Rice, *The Winning Side: Questions on Living the Culture of Life* (2000), 243–55.

40. Address of Pope John Paul II to the Plenary Assembly of the Pontifical Council for Culture, March 16, 2002.

41. See *Redemptoris Missio, The Mission of the Redeemer* (1990), no. 86.

6

The Public Morality of Having Children

Gerard V. Bradley

Some people are puzzled by the tendency of moral traditionalists to object on moral grounds to the production of human beings by in vitro fertilization. After all, moral tradition strongly affirms the goodness of transmitting life to new persons. Why, then, should couples who are incapable of begetting children in acts of marital intercourse not resort to in vitro processes in order to become parents? The short answer is that the manufacturing of children is inconsistent with respect for their basic equality and human dignity.

Children are to be desired under a description that does not reduce the child to the status of a product to be brought into existence at its parents' will and for their ends. Children rather are to be treated as persons—possessing full human dignity—which the spouses are eager to welcome (and take responsibility for) as a perfective participant in the community established by their marriage (i.e., their family). (It is in this sense that one speaks of children as "gifts" that "supervene" on marital acts.) This is not to suggest that there is anything wrong with spouses engaging in marital intercourse because they "want" a child. It is merely to indicate the description under which the "wanting" of the child is consistent with his or her dignity as a person, and to highlight the fact that the marital significance of properly motivated spousal intercourse obtains whether or not conception is hoped for, results, or is even possible. Importantly, however, the intrinsic worth and dignity of a child is in no way diminished by any moral defect in the act that brings that child into existence.

In my view, children conceived in marital intercourse participate in the good of their parents' marriage and are themselves non-instrumental aspects of its perfection; thus, spouses rightly hope for and welcome children, not as "products" they "make," but rather, as gifts, which if all goes well, supervene on their acts on marital union. This understanding of children as gifts to be accepted and valued for their own sake—rather than as objects that may be willed and brought into being for one's own purposes—obviously coheres well with certain theistic metaphysical views, including Jewish and Christian views. It can, however, also be accommodated by Buddhist and certain other non-theistic views. Some understanding along these lines of the moral relationship of parents to the children they may conceive is essential to the rational affirmation of the dignity of children as persons: i.e., as ends in themselves, and not mere means of satisfying desires of their parents; as subjects of justice (including fundamental and inviolable human rights), rather than objects of will. Alternative understandings run into severe difficulties in explaining why children may not properly be understood—and rightly treated —as the property of their parents.

It seems to me, then, and I submit to you, that the relevant task of a sound public morality is to support and maintain marriage as the uniquely appropriate context for having and raising children. A sound public morality would, most notably, not recognize same-sex relationships as marriages, or as its legal equivalent under another name.

In the balance of this paper, I try to explain why marriage deserves the protection of public authority which it has long enjoyed, and why same-sex couples cannot marry.

LAW AND THE CULTURE OF MARRIAGE

Marriage is truly the state's business, even though it is not the state's creation. Civil law must often, for the sake of persons' flourishing, enter into creative partnerships with institutions and practices it does not make—at least where those institutions contribute to the common good and where they need law's help to prosper. Public authority helps in various ways—it recognizes, ratifies, regulates, promotes, supports, and protects. Law supervenes upon these institutions, and by so doing creates, within limits, a legal version or dimension of a particular social practice or institution. The state's support of marriage and family is the most important such partnership.

The partnership is quite one-sided: law exists for these institutions because law is for the persons whose well-being and flourishing is dependent upon them. Marriage does not exist for law, or for the polity, or for the success of the nation-state as a world historical actor, or for the GNP. Things are the other way round. Law is to support certain institutions of civil society for the sake of the common good.

Does marriage need law's help? Yes. People are not free to choose the culture in which they live, interact, court, marry, make love, have children. One set of laws shapes, structures, and ultimately holds in place by legal sanction the public architecture and, in great measure, the cultural forms of these practices and relationships. As legal philosopher Joseph Raz says, "monogamy, assuming that it is the only valuable form of marriage, cannot be practiced by an individual. It requires a culture which recognizes it, and which supports it through the public's attitude and through its formal institutions."[1]

Raz does not suppose that, in a culture whose law and public morality do not support monogamy, someone who happens to believe in it somehow will be unable to restrict himself to having one wife or will be required to take additional wives. His point, as expressed by Princeton's Robert George, is rather that "even if monogamy is a key element of a sound understanding of marriage, large numbers of people will fail to understand that or why that is the case—and will therefore fail to grasp the value of monogamy and the intelligible point of practicing it—unless they are assisted by a culture which supports monogamous marriage. Marriage is the type of good which can be participated in, or fully participated in, only by people who properly understand it and choose it with a proper understanding in mind; yet people's ability to properly understand it, and thus to choose it, depends upon institutions and cultural understandings that transcend individual choice."[2]

Marriage is thus both "hard" and "soft". Marriage is "hard" in that its constitutive features are beyond human choosing. Marriage is "soft" in that persons can only marry according to the "marriage" made available to them. William cannot marry his male neighbor or the two sisters next door, for neither same-sex marriage nor polygamy is, in truth, possible. This "hard" moral reality enjoys public recognition and support. Public authority in America has always protected, often through criminal penalties, the constitutive features of marriage: monogamous, heterosexual, sexually exclusive, the legitimate context for having children.

Same-sex marriage has always been legally impossible: unlike, say, robbery and jaywalking, acts which persons are capable of committing but which the state prohibits, same-sex marriage was not so much prohibited as it was thought to be impossible. Everyone understands that one is able to choose to kill. It is just that no one should. But the legal unavailability of same-sex marriage has always been understood as a reflection of the nature of marriage. (Only recently has it been branded by advocates of same-sex unions as the raw preference of a benighted majority.)

Marriage is nevertheless "soft" (malleable, subjective), too. As George and Raz both suggest, someone entering into marriage can only choose what he or she understands marriage to be. (This is an example of a wider truth about human choosing and acting: no one can choose an option which is never presented to the mind or to the will for decision.) Someone who chooses to marry for life, to the exclusion of sex with all others, simply enters into a different relationship than someone who does not really choose fidelity unto death. Similarly, someone who enters into a marriage understanding it as procreative enters into a different relationship from one who does not.

The "marriage" available in any society is powerfully formed by law, and by culture (itself shaped by law). All too often, corrupt culture and law conspire to deprive people of the opportunity to choose (real) marriage— where, for example, polygamy is the social norm, or where wives are treated as chattel, and not as equal spouses. Does anyone doubt that the moral acceptability of interracial marriage changed (for the good) when the law changed, when interracial couples became legally able to marry?

Someone might object: the civil law does not require married couples to have children. Infertile couples have always been able to marry. Today many couples marry without a firm intention to have children and some marrying couples are known to be sterile. As an Indiana court recently said, "not all opposite-sex couples may be able to reproduce on their own, or may wish to have children at all"[3]. These considerations lie behind Justice Scalia's point (expressed in Lawrence v. Texas) that procreation cannot be the reason why the civil law limits marriage to man and woman. If, then, procreation is not the law's end, why exactly is marriage impossible for two men?

The state does not inquire of every opposite-sex couple concerning their ability or intent to procreate. The state is not required to deny sterile couples the opportunity to marry. Neither sound reasoning nor our law requires that every marriage actually be fruitful. The exact intentions of men and women marrying, their decisions later about the number and spacing of children, the marital bedroom—and indeed the whole family's life (within broad limits) are private –none of the state's business. The state does enough, but no more than it must, in witnessing to the truth about marriage by limiting it to the union of man and woman.

Legal recognition of same-sex marriage would not signal to our country's (young) people (especially) that their government has reconsidered some matter of policy, has recalculated costs and benefits, has acted upon new information or the latest techniques—and changed its mind about some regulation. Recognizing same-sex marriage would instead be a state broadcast of a new (putative) truth about marriage (correcting an ancient prejudice, or lie): marriage is not really ordered to procreation. What was off the menu of available options is now on it. What could not be chosen, now can be. Culture, popular practice, and individual choices—the whole reality of marriage on offer in the state—is thus transformed.

The U.S. Supreme Court knows this profound capacity of law to shape an entire culture. Affirming the central holding of Roe v. Wade the Court wrote in Planned Parenthood v. Casey that "[a]n entire generation has come of age free to assume Roe's concept of liberty in defining the capacity of woman to act in society, and to make reproductive decisions."[4] With what effect? "[F]or two decades . . . people have organized intimate relationships and made choices that define their views of themselves and their places in society, in reliance on the availability of abortion in the event that contraception should fail. The ability of women to participate equally in the economic and social life of the Nation has been facilitated by their ability to control their reproductive lives."[5]

Note well: Casey was not talking about just, or even mainly, the millions of women who had abortions. The Court was talking about how Roe altered the psychology and self-understanding, the dreams and achievements, of every woman. All women, according to the Court, enjoy the benefits of ultimate control over their reproductive lives: legal abortion like unemployment insurance or Medicaid, or any other strand in the social safety net. No matter what chances one takes with one's money or job, no matter how bad one's luck turns, one knows that one is not going to starve, or be left to die with no doctor to lend a hand. According to the land's highest court, then, Roe would have transformed our world even if no one actually had an abortion.

Legally recognizing same-sex "marriage" will reconstitute our world of marriage and family. No one can say with confidence how rapidly the legal revolution will trickle down to ordinary persons' understanding of marriage, and alter what marriage is, to them and for them. But the abortion example, the lessons of history, and the warnings of keen observers such as Joseph Raz all give us reason to fear that the descent could be both fast and steep.

It will also be unprecedented, for even those Supreme Court decisions which, as it turns out, are claimed to stand for broad sexual freedom, do not.

To these leading constitutional cases I turn.

THE CONSTITUTIONAL TRADITION OF MARRIAGE

In Griswold v. Connecticut, 381 U.S. 479, 486 (1965), the United States Supreme Court described "a right of privacy older than the Bill of Rights", that surrounding husband and wife:

> Marriage is a coming together for better or for worse, hopefully enduring, and intimate to the degree of being sacred. . . . [I]t is an association for as noble a purpose as any involved in our prior decisions.

Griswold involved a statute that criminalized a married couple's use of contraceptives. But the Griswold Court articulated a broader, encompassing immunity. Griswold's "marital privacy" was (as Justice White said in his concurrence) the "right to be free of regulation of the intimacies of the marriage relationship." Justice Douglas asked in his opinion for the Court, "[w]ould we allow the police to search the sacred precincts of marital bedrooms for telltale signs of the use of contraceptives?" Of course, neither the location nor the dimensions of a couple's bedroom makes it "sacred." No judge would hesitate, for example, to authorize a search of a whole home for bomb residue, stolen goods, drugs, or weapons. The force of Justice Douglas's question is carried by the implicit reference to what a married couple, as such, characteristically does in their bedroom.

The Griswold opinions steadily refer to the marital "relationship," to marital "privacy," and to marital "intimacy" (and "intimacies"). The Court's explicit focus was not a particular sex act or contraceptives as such. The majority opinions even abstain from express judgments—favorable or unfavorable—about the moral worth of contraception. Griswold is best understood as standing for the married couple's right of non-interference, or immunity, for all their consensual, private sexual acts.

Griswold recognized the unique—"sacred"—place of marital sexual intimacies in our constitutional order. Being "sacred" means that they are beyond state interference or regulation. This elevated station implies that non- and extra-marital sexual acts stand on a different, more prosaic footing. They are open to state regulation.

In his 1961 Poe v. Ullman dissent (which on the merits anticipated the Court's holding in Griswold), Justice Harlan agreed that marriage is the distinguishing principle of sexual morality, and elaborated its implications:

> The laws regarding marriage which provide both when the sexual powers may be used and the legal and societal context in which children are born and brought up, as well as laws forbidding adultery, fornication and homosexual practices, which express the negative of the proposition, confining sexuality to lawful marriage, a pattern deeply pressed into the substance of our social life. . . .

The teaching of Griswold and Poe is this—the State is authorized by the Constitution, and required by the common good, to promote marriage by: respecting the privacy of the marital bedroom, and by discouraging sexual acts outside of marriage. The State's discouragement of fornication, homosexual acts, and other non-marital sexual activity may and commonly has (as Justice Harlan said) included making crimes of some, or all, of those acts.

Justice Harlan indicated why treating the deviant acts of unmarried persons as crimes does not impose an arbitrary, majoritarian morality upon an oppressed minority. The discouragement arises not from a paternalistic desire to correct and punish persons for their sexual misbehavior for the sake of their moral improvement. Much less does it arise from a dislike for the persons who would engage in deviate acts, same-sex or otherwise. The State's discouragement of non- and extra-marital sexual acts is a requirement of the great common (and thus objective) good of marriage.

Some people say that, in a diverse society such as our own, the civil institution of marriage should swing free from all moral conceptions of it, even if those conceptions are accepted (for sake of argument) as objective, and even true. The idea might be to expand, or flatten out, the legal contours of marriage, so as to make it available to everyone on their own terms. The idea might be, in other words, to privatize marriage.

This suggestion must be rejected. In the first place, one might well wonder about the intelligibility of "privatized" civil marriage. Second, the suggestion is utterly incompatible with our whole constitutional, legal and cultural tradition, which (as Griswold shows) has sought to promote and sustain marriage as a great common good. Finally, the aspiration to a value-free marital regime is impossible. If the opposite-sex character of marriage depends upon an illicit moral view, why not monogamy, too? Upon what proper basis is marriage limited to two persons, or three, or four? Upon what proper basis could any presumption of sexual fidelity and permanence be grounded? "Value-free" marriage would turn out to be nothing at all.

Now, in Eisenstadt v. Baird, a four-Justice majority of the Court stated that "whatever the rights of the individual to access to contraceptives may be, the rights must be the same for the unmarried and the married alike." The Eisenstadt Court supported this conclusion by disaggregating the married couple. The Eisenstadt Court said:

> [T]he marital couple . . . is an association of two individuals each with a separate intellectual and emotional makeup. If the right of privacy means anything, it is the right of the individual, married or single, to be free from unwarranted governmental intrusion into matters so fundamentally affecting a person as the decision whether to bear or beget a child.

Eisenstadt could be said to warrant acceptance of some constitutional right to sexual freedom. The reasoning might be stated as follows: "if the right of privacy means anything, it is the right of individuals to be free of governmental regulation of sexual acts between, or among, consenting adults, at least when the acts occur in private."

Not so. The reasoning of Eisenstadt offers no support for extending the disaggregation of marriage into the whole realm of sexual conduct, and the opinion expressly contradicts such an extension.

Eisenstadt focused on the reproductive consequences of sexual intercourse between unmarried men and women. The Justices aimed to prevent the State from "punishing" fornicators with maternity or paternity. The Court referred throughout not to singles' deviant sexual acts, but to "sexual intercourse" and procreative "sexual relations." Eisenstadt stands, after all, for an individual's privacy regarding the "bear[ing] or beget[ting of] a child", though "bear" amounted to dictum (no question of an already pregnant woman's options was presented to the Eisenstadt Court). The dictum became law within a year. It is Roe to which Eisenstadt pointed, not to a liberationist ethic of sexual acts.

Besides, Eisenstadt expressly said that non- and extramarital sexual acts were "evils" (the Court's word), against which States possess a "full measure of discretion in fashioning means to prevent." Eisenstadt did not simply grant this discretion, nor did it label fornication "evil" for argument's sake. Eisenstadt instead explicitly

> conced[ed] that the State could, consistently with the Equal Protection Clause, regard the problems of extramarital and premarital sexual relations as "evils . . . of different dimensions and proportions, requiring difficult remedies."

The Eisenstadt Court recognized, too, that reasonable and constitutionally permissible attempts to deter fornication and adultery could include making those acts criminal. Eisenstadt does not stand for a broad right of individual sexual freedom. It affirms instead the States' traditional authority to promote marriage by deterring—even by criminal sanctions—all sexual acts outside of marriage.

MARRIAGE AND THE COMMON GOOD

We have seen that marriage needs law's help. How does marriage contribute to the political common good? More exactly, how does the procreative orientation of marriage benefit the polity?

The unique appropriateness of marriage as the context for having children does not depend upon a raw societal interest in population replacement. It is not a matter of having a pro-natalist legislative policy. This unique appropriateness does not depend upon statistical verification of claims about children's grades, emotional adjustment, or some other measure of social well being when they live in traditional mother and father homes. Likewise, the imprudence of public policies encouraging the formation of families headed by same-sex couples does not depend upon claims about the comparative disadvantages—by the same statistical measures—of such households as environments for raising children.

This unique appropriateness is not about social scientific findings at all. It has rather to do with the valuable human relationships which the reproductive union of man and woman makes possible: the married couple (as husband and wife; mother and father); father and daughter; father and son; between mother and daughter, mother and son.

This complementarity goes well beyond the biological unity possible for man and woman. It is, however, partly that. By their marital acts the couple actualize, or express, in a profound and special way their whole married life together. When their marital acts bear the fruit of children, these children are (literally, then) the issue of their marriage: embodiments and thereby extensions, into space and time, of their parents' marriage. Mother and father are equally, and exclusively, parents of all their children. All the children are, one compared to the others, equally and wholly the offspring of the same parents. This family-wide equality, mutuality and natural bond of identity is the wellspring and ground of love, duty, loyalty, and care-giving—the whole matrix of family life. Nothing can replace it.

This complementarity is partly psychological. It results in a unique combination of male and female psyches, temperaments and culturally shaped roles for the husband/father, wife/mother, daughter/sister, son/brother. One need not and we do not endorse all features of our culture's—or any culture's—gender role definition. But some such rough definition and differentiation according to gender is found in every culture, for some such differentiation is endemic to our experience of life as embodied males or females.

No society's conception of how a husband, or an eldest daughter, for example, is to behave is beyond criticism. But being a wife and mother is scarcely a matter of assuming a socially constructed type. It is a natural moral reality upon which culture—and law—rightly supervene, and in so doing structure, specify, reinforce, protect. And in doing that culture—and law— promote these great (natural, morally valuable) opportunities for human flourishing, keeping them alive, intact, and available for choice by persons within the culture.

These marital and familial relationships form the great moral reality which drives the law's protection of marriage as the morally appropriate context of parenting. This factor is no more subtle or beyond the state's concern than is the correct judgment that the factor of equality of marital friendship lies at, or very near, the heart of the state's legitimate judgment that polygamy is not supportable, even to the point of making criminal a person's attempts (indeed, rendering their acts merely attempts) at plural marriage.

PLURAL MARRIAGE?

Once marriage is no longer a bodily communion oriented towards procreation then three or more persons could as readily constitute a marriage as could two. As an Indiana court recently said, "[t]here is no inherent reason why [Plaintiff's] theories, including the encouragement of long-term stable relationships, the sharing of economic lives, the enhancement of emotional well-being . . . could not be applied to groups of three or more."[6] In this scenario, the underlying, unavoidable equality and mutuality of the traditional family is out the window.

Marriage is, and has always been understood by our law to be, a bodily, two-in-one flesh union of persons. That is why it is impossible for two men or two women to marry: it is impossible for them to enter into bodily communion. Apart from this understanding of marriage, the legal requirement of consummation (which is only fulfilled by vaginal intercourse) is unintelligible. Apart from this understanding of marriage, there cannot be any sense in which marriage is characteristically procreative, or intrinsically ordered to having and raising children.

If marriage is understood, however, as an association of individuals who seek from each other and from their relationship certain emotional, sexual, psychological satisfactions, and who set up a household with pooled finances, the ineligibility of same-sex couples to wed surely appears unreasoned, and arbitrary. Where marriage is stripped of its meaning as an integral, bodily union oriented in some sense towards procreation, there indeed appears to be no reason why same-sex couples may not marry.

Legal recognition of same-sex relationships as marriages would, therefore, imply the law's redefinition of "marriage," not a subtle expansion of eligibility. This redefinition—that marriage is not a bodily or two-in-one communion between persons of the opposite sex—would be so extraordinary and unprecedented that it would mean the end of marriage as the law, and the overwhelming majority of Americans, has always understood it. The new relationship might take the place of "marriage" in the law books. But in truth, and to almost all Americans, it would not be marriage at all. It would instead be more the sexually involved relationship of householders.

And there would, then, be no non-arbitrary basis whatsoever upon which monogamy could be legally maintained. This Supreme Court recognized keenly near the end of the last century that marriage, being a two-in-one communion, simply could not be polygamous. Notwithstanding the sincere beliefs of many people in Mormon communities in plural marriage, the fact was—and is—that marriage is for one man and one woman. One need not agree with all the measures that Congress took, and that the Court approved, to preserve marriage in Utah to see that fundamentally the effort was sound, and right.

CONCLUSION

Some critics of the view I have defended here assert that it relegates, at least by implication, homosexuals to second-class citizenship. This criticism is wide of the mark. The truth is that homosexuality is irrelevant to almost every question pertaining to the common good of political society. That is partly because the most important civil rights are human rights. Human rights attach to everyone because they are human persons. These rights do not acquire their sense, and vary not at all in their precise content, according upon one's "sexual orientation," or, for that matter, on the state of one's character in regard to other matters, such as justice.

Homosexuality is almost entirely irrelevant partly because people are to be morally judged on the basis of their conduct not their condition. Simply being homosexual is not, and should not be, the basis of criminal liability because being homosexual is not an act. Similarly, it is wrong to think of "punishing" (a moral category) anyone for being homosexual, or for any other unjust attitude or desire.

Finally, homosexuality is almost entirely irrelevant because most of the particular rights and duties of political and civil life do not implicate one's sexual activity, habits or orientation—whatever it is. Eligibility for drivers licenses, for library privileges, to sit as jurors; duties to pay taxes, observe the speed limit, and to avoid harms to others have their sources in skills, opportunities and moral norms which do not include sexual inclination or activity in any way, for anyone. "Heterosexuals" (as such) are no more, and no less eligible, for jury service than "homosexuals" (as such) are.

The law does not condemn homosexuals to loneliness, nor does it discriminate against same-sex friendship. The law has always regarded genuine friendship, apart from family ties and sexual intimacy, as good grounds for some legal relations. Any two people can sign a lease or take out a loan. Anyone may be given power of attorney, be appointed guardian ad litem, executor of an estate. The law presumes that trusted others—friends—will fill such important legal slots. Friendship therefore has a vital place in the good life, a place recognized and facilitated by our law.

Marriage, it is true, is a type of friendship. But, marriage is a unique type of friendship, specified by the capacity to engage in reproductive type acts, and it is simply unavailable to same-sex couples.

NOTES

1. J. Raz, *The Morality of Freedom*, 162 (1986)

2. "'Same-sex Marriage' and 'Moral Neutrality'", K. Whitehead, ed., *Marriage and the Common Good*, 93 (2001).

3. *Morrison v. Sadler, Marion County Court (slip opinion), May 7, 2003.*

4. 505 U.S. 833, 860 (1992)

5. 505 U.S. at 856.

6. *Morrison, supra* note 10, at 13.

Index

Index

Contributors

Gerard Bradley, JD is Professor of Law at the University of Notre Dame, where he has taught since 1992. During the Fall of 2001, he was Visiting Professor of Law at Ave Maria School of Law in Ann Arbor, Michigan. He taught at the University of Illinois College of Law from 1983 until 1992. Professor Bradley has published widely in the fields of constitutional law, legal philosophy, and on subjects at the intersection of law and morality. He has testified before Congressional committees on many occasions, including testimony on cloning and abortion-related issues. From 1995 until 2001, Professor Bradley served as President of the Fellowship of Catholic Scholars.

Jean Bethke Elshtain, PhD is the Laura Spelman Rockefeller Professor of Social and Political Ethics at the University of Chicago. She is the author or editor of many books including: *Public Man, Private Woman: Woman in Social and Political Thought, Meditations on Modern Political Thought, Democracy on Trial, Politics and the Human Body* and *Just War Theory.* Dr. Elshtain is also the author of over four hundred articles and essays in scholarly journals and journals of civic opinion. In 1996, she was elected a Fellow of the American Academy of Arts and Sciences. She is the recipient of seven honorary degrees and co-director of the recently established Pew Forum on Religion and American Public Life.

Francis Cardinal George, O.M.I. is the archbishop of the city of Chicago. He entered the Missionary Oblates of Mary Immaculate in 1957 and was ordained a priest on December 21, 1963. Cardinal George has served as Bishop in the diocese of Yakima and as Archbishop in the city of Portland. He was installed as Archbishop of Chicago on May 27, 1996 and named Cardinal by Pope John Paul II January 18, 1998.

Peter J. Kreeft, PhD is Professor of Philosophy at Boston College. He received his MA in 1961 and PhD in 1965 from Fordham University, and pursued his post-graduate study at Yale University. He has taught for over forty years. He has accumulated several awards and honors, including the Woodrow Wilson Fellowship, Yale-Sterling Fellowship, Newman Alumni Scholarship, Danforth Asian Religions Fellowship, and the Weathersfield Homeland Foundation Fellowship. He is a regular contributor to several Christian publications and is the author of over 40 books including *Three Philosophies of Life, Prayer: the Great Conversation*, and *Fundamentals of the Faith*.

Patrick Lee, PhD is professor of philosophy at the Franciscan University of Steubenville. He grew up in Dallas Texas, received his B.A. from the University of Dallas in 1974, his M.A. in philosophy from Niagara University in 1977, and his PhD in philosophy from Marquette University in 1980. He is a specialist in ethics and in the philosophy of St. Thomas Aquinas. He has published articles in various scholarly journals, such *as American Catholic Philosophical Quarterly, International Philosophical Quarterly*, and *Faith and Philosophy*. His book, *Abortion and Unborn Human Life,* appeared in 1996 and is available from Catholic University of America Press or from Amazon.com. He is now working on a book together with Robert P. George tentatively titled, "Dualism and Contemporary Ethical Issues."

Nicholas C. Lund-Molfese, MA, JD is the director of the Integritas Institute at the University of Illinois at Chicago and the coordinator of the Ministry in Higher Education Agency of the Archdiocese of Chicago. Mr. Lund-Molfese received his JD and MA in philosophy from the University of Illinois. He is the co-editor of the book *Human Dignity and Reproductive Technology* (University Press of America; spring 2004) and has authored scholarly articles in journals such as the *Catholic Social Science Review, The American Journal of Jurisprudence*, and *The American Journal of Bioethics*.

Charles E. Rice, JD is Professor Emeritus of Law at the University of Notre Dame Law School and Visiting Professor of Law at Ave Maria School of Law, Ann Arbor, Michigan. His areas of specialization are constitutional law, jurisprudence, and torts. He now teaches Jurisprudence in the fall term at Ave Maria and in the spring term at Notre Dame. He received his BA from the College of the Holy Cross, his JD from Boston College Law School, and the LLM and JSD from New York University. He served in the Marine Corps and is a Lt. Col. in the U.S. Marine Corps Reserve. He practiced law in New York City and taught at New York University Law School and Fordham Law School before joining, in 1969, the faculty of law at Notre Dame. He served for eight years as State Vice-Chairman of the New York State Conservative Party, and he has played a role in many other organizations.